100 Medical Emergencies for Finals

Prasanna Sooriakumaran
Specialist Registrar in Urology
South Thames Deanery

Channa Jayasena
Specialist Registrar in Diabetes and Endocrinology
Hammersmith Hospital, London

and

Anjla Sharman
Clinical Lecturer in the Division of Primary Care
University of Nottingham, and
General Practitioner, Nottingham

Foreword by
Ruth Brown
Consultant in A&E Medicine
St Mary's Hospital, London

Radcliffe Publishing
Oxford ● Seattle

Radcliffe Publishing Ltd
18 Marcham Road
Abingdon
Oxon OX14 1AA
United Kingdom

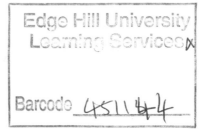

www.radcliffe-oxford.com
Electronic catalogue and worldwide online ordering facility.

British Library Cataloguing in Publication Data

A catalogue record for this book is available from the British Library.

ISBN-10: 1 85775 747 5
ISBN-13: 978 1 85775 747 7

Typeset by Advance Typesetting Ltd, Oxford
Printed and bound by TJ International Ltd, Padstow, Cornwall

Contents

Foreword   vii

Preface   ix

About the authors   x

Acknowledgements   xi

List of abbreviations   xii

1   Cardiac conditions   1
    Basic life support   1
    Cardiac arrest: ventricular fibrillation   5
    Cardiac arrest: pulseless electrical activity   8
    Cardiac arrest: asystole   11
    Acute coronary syndrome   13
    Narrow complex tachycardia   17
    Broad complex tachycardia   20
    Bradycardia   22
    Acute pulmonary oedema   25
    Malignant hypertension   27
    Cardiac tamponade   29

2   Respiratory conditions   31
    Acute asthma   31
    Acute exacerbation of chronic obstructive
        pulmonary disease   35
    Pneumothorax   39

3   Neurology   43
    Coma/reduced consciousness   43
    Raised intracranial pressure   46
    Meningitis   48
    Stroke   51
    Cerebral haemorrhage   54
    Status epilepticus   56

4   Renal conditions   59
    Acute renal failure   59
    Hyperkalaemia   62
    Rhabdomyolysis   64

5   Endocrine conditions   66
    Diabetic ketoacidosis   66
    Hyper-osmolar non-ketotic acidosis   70
    Hypoglycaemia   74
    Phaeochromocytoma   76
    Addisonian crisis   78

6   Haematology/oncology   81
    Deep vein thrombosis   81
    Pulmonary embolism   83
    Disseminated intravascular coagulopathy   86
    Neutropenic sepsis   88
    Sickle-cell crisis   91
    Acute transfusion reaction   94
    Superior vena caval obstruction   97

7   Abdominal conditions   99
    Appendicitis   99
    Acute pancreatitis   102
    Ascending cholangitis   106
    Acute peritonitis   107
    Liver failure   110
    Large bowel obstruction   114
    Small bowel obstruction   117
    Mesenteric ischaemia and infarction   118
    Strangulated hernia   119
    Upper gastrointestinal bleeding   121
    Lower gastrointestinal bleeding   124

8   Urology   126
    Testicular torsion   126
    Ureteric colic   128
    Acute retention of urine   130

Acute pyelonephritis   132
Priapism   133

9 Vascular conditions   134
Ruptured abdominal aortic aneurysm   134
Aortic dissection   136
Acute limb ischaemia   139

10 Orthopaedics   141
Fractures   141
Spinal injuries   143
Cauda equina syndrome   145
Compartment syndrome   146
Acutely inflamed joint   148

11 Trauma   149
Trauma: general principles   149
Trauma: airway   152
Trauma: breathing   154
Trauma: circulation   156
Head injury   158
Drowning and hypothermia   161

12 Plastic surgery/dermatology   165
Burns   165
Wounds   169
Erythroderma   171
Stevens–Johnson's syndrome   173

13 Ophthalmology/otorhinolaryngology   176
Red eye   176
Sudden loss of vision   179
Maxillofacial trauma   182
Epistaxis   185

14 Paediatrics   187
Stridor   187
Febrile convulsions   190
Pyloric stenosis   192

Non-accidental injury 194
Paediatric trauma and resuscitation 197

15 Obstetrics/gynaecology **201**
Ectopic pregnancy 201
Placenta praevia 204
Placental abruption 206
Pre-eclampsia 208
Cord prolapse 211
Shoulder dystocia 213
Postpartum haemorrhage 215
Toxic shock syndrome 218

16 Psychiatric conditions **221**
Acute psychosis: assessment 221
Acute psychosis: management 225
Deliberate self-harm and suicide 228
Delirium 231
Alcohol withdrawal 235

17 Toxicology **237**
Paracetamol overdose 237
Salicylate poisoning 241
Opiate overdose 244
Tricyclic antidepressant overdose 246

18 Miscellaneous conditions **250**
Shock 250
Sepsis and its sequelae 253
Anaphylaxis 258
Post-operative pyrexia 260
Acute pain management 264

Index **267**

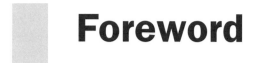

Foreword

For medical students and MMC Foundation Programme doctors, acute emergencies may present the most challenging and stressful events in their careers so far. Acquiring the knowledge and competences to manage those emergencies requires a different approach to standard medical teaching and study. Current undergraduate medical education, with its emphasis on the whole patient pathway, communication skills and self-directed learning, inevitably leaves gaps in the learner's knowledge about the practicalities of treatment or produces formulaic (ABC) solutions that do not go far enough in the real situation. The foundation years are designed to enable doctors to acquire competences in acute presentations, and embrace assessment of those competences. However, the availability of easily digested and clear advice on emergencies is limited, and inconsistent.

For those preparing to work in the emergency environment or to answer examination questions on those cases, this book is an ideal source for simple and focused advice. Many emergency medicine textbooks provide comprehensive reviews of a clinical topic, in great detail and across a broad spread of conditions. The selection of the top 100 topics in this book reflects the case mix in the average emergency department or hospital ward base. The easy-to-access, clearly defined sections within each topic, provide practical advice and limited but selected further reading opportunities. Use of simple algorithms and flow charts assist the development of skills in decision making or skills in the selection of discriminatory tests. The design and layout means it is easy to dip in and out of, either as part of revision for exams, as easy reading in short bursts, or as an aide-mémoire in the emergency department. As such it might well appeal to other healthcare professionals, for example the emergency nurse practitioner or pre-hospital personnel.

The three authors' differing career paths and specialty selection mean the book has an authority derived from their respective areas of expertise. By combining their experience they have produced a useful handbook for the development of practical approaches to emergencies, whether for examination purposes or the early years of medical practice.

Dr Ruth Brown FRCS, FFAEM
Consultant in Accident & Emergency Medicine
St Mary's Hospital, London
February 2006

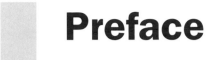

Preface

Medical students need to assimilate a vast amount of information as they approach their final examinations. However, the topic they most frequently encounter in examinations, in both multiple-choice and viva formats, is the recognition and management of emergencies. After all, as junior doctors they must be able to deal promptly with these conditions, above all others. The aim of this book is to give clinical medical students the basics of the major emergency conditions that they may encounter, both in final examinations and on the wards as a foundation-year doctor. We have attempted to make the book easy to read, and have added snippets of the relevant basic sciences as appropriate in order to aid understanding of the principles involved. Medical emergencies across all of the major specialties are covered, and we envisage that this book will also be of use to more senior doctors as a quick revision guide during preparation for their specialty examinations.

P Sooriakumaran
C Jayasena
A Sharman
February 2006

About the authors

Prasanna Sooriakumaran BMedSci (Hons), BMBS (Hons), MRCS (Eng) graduated with Honours from the University of Nottingham, and is currently a Specialist Registrar in Urology finishing off his PhD in Prostate Cancer. He has previously been an Anatomy Demonstrator, SSM Tutor, Finals Tutor and Education Coordinator for numerous medical students in London. He is the co-coordinator of the trainees' advisory group of the international campaign to revitalise academic medicine, a peer reviewer for many international journals and publishers, and has won six postgraduate prizes, written one other book *Key Topics in Human Diseases*, two book chapters and over 100 papers and abstracts in peer-reviewed journals.

Channa Jayasena MA, MB, BChir, MRCP obtained a double-first degree in developmental and neural biology and a medical degree from Cambridge University. He is currently a specialist registrar in endocrinology and metabolism at Hammersmith Hospital, London. As well as teaching on two MRCP clinical courses, he is a clinical finals tutor and BSc supervisor at Imperial College, London. He has also been an undergraduate college supervisor at Cambridge University.

Anjla Sharman BMedSci (Hons), BMBS, DFFP, DRCOG, MRCGP (Distinction) obtained her degrees in medical sciences and medicine from the University of Nottingham, and is currently studying for a Masters degree in medical education. She recently completed her vocational training and now combines work as a part-time GP with her post as a clinical lecturer in the Division of Primary Care at the University of Nottingham. She is also a clinical supervisor for GP registrars at Nottingham Emergency Medical Services, and she organises an MRCGP Preparation Course.

Acknowledgements

We would like to thank our own clinical teachers, past and present, for their words of wisdom which have been incorporated in this book. We are grateful to the staff at Radcliffe Publishing Ltd, in particular Mr Andrew Bax, for their continued support.

Most of all, we would like to thank the numerous medical students, especially those at the University of Nottingham and at medical schools of the University of London, for providing the inspiration for this work.

List of abbreviations

ABG	Arterial blood gases
ACE	Angiotensin-converting enzyme
ACS	Acute coronary syndrome
ACTH	Adrenocorticotropic hormone
AF	Atrial fibrillation
AIDS	Acquired immunodeficiency syndrome
ALT	Alanine aminotransferase
AMD	Age-related macular degeneration
APTT	Activated partial thromboplastin time
ARDS	Acute respiratory distress syndrome
ARF	Acute renal failure
AST	Aspartate aminotransferase
ASW	Approved social worker
ATLS	Advanced Trauma Life Support
AV	Atrioventricular
AXR	Abdominal X-ray
BIH	Benign intracranial hypertension
BLS	Basic life support
BM	Blood glucose monitoring
BP	Blood pressure
CAPD	Chronic ambulatory peritoneal dialysis
CBD	Common bile duct
CK	Creatine kinase
CNS	Central nervous system
COPD	Chronic obstructive pulmonary disease
CPAP	Continuous positive airways pressure
CPR	Cardiopulmonary resuscitation
CRP	C-reactive protein
CSF	Cerebrospinal fluid
CT	Computed tomography

CTG	Cardiotopography
CVP	Central venous pressure
CXR	Chest X-ray
DC	Direct current
DIC	Disseminated intravascular coagulation
DKA	Diabetic ketoacidosis
DRE	Digital rectal examination
ECG	Electrocardiogram
EMD	Electromechanical dissociation
ERCP	Endoscopic retrograde cholangiopancreatography
ESR	Erythrocyte sedimentation rate
ESWL	Extra-corporeal shock-wave lithotripsy
FBC	Full blood count
G&S	Group and save
GA	General anaesthesia
GCS	Glasgow Coma Scale
GI	Gastrointestinal
GTN	Glyceryl trinitrate
Hb	Haemoglobin
HCG	Human chorionic gonadotropin
HDU	High-dependency unit
HIV	Human immunodeficiency virus
HONK	Hyper-osmolar non-ketotic acidosis
ICP	Intracranial pressure
IM	Intramuscular
INR	International normalised ratio
ITU	Intensive-therapy unit
IUGR	Intrauterine growth retardation
IV	Intravenous
IVU	Intravenous urogram
JVP	Jugulovenous pressure
KUB	Kidney, ureters and bladder X-ray
LA	Local anaesthesia
LBBB	Left bundle branch block
LDH	Lactate dehydrogenase
LFTs	Liver function tests
MI	Myocardial infarction
MRI	Magnetic resonance imaging

MS	Multiple sclerosis
MSU	Midstream urine
NBM	Nil by mouth
NG	Nasogastric
NIV	Non-invasive ventilation
NSAIDs	Non-steroidal anti-inflammatory drugs
OCP	Oral contraceptive pill
OGD	Oesophago-gastro-duodenoscopy
pCO_2	Partial pressure of carbon dioxide
pO_2	Partial pressure of oxygen
PEA	Pulseless electrical activity
PEF	Peak expiratory flow
PR	Per rectum
PT	Prothrombin time
PTC	Percutaneous transhepatic cholangiography
PUJ	Pelvi-ureteric junction
RIF	Right iliac fossa
RMN	Registered mental health nurse
RR	Respiratory rate
SAH	Subarachnoid haemorrhage
SaO_2	Oxygen saturation
SLE	Systemic lupus erythematosus
SOB	Shortness of breath
SVT	Supraventricular tachycardia
TFTs	Thyroid function tests
TIA	Transient ischaemic attack
TPA	Tissue plasminogen activator
TPN	Total parenteral nutrition
TSS	Toxic shock syndrome
TTE	Transthoracic echocardiography
TURP	Transurethral resection of the prostate
U&Es	Urea and electrolytes
US	Ultrasound
UTI	Urinary tract infection
VF	Ventricular fibrillation
VT	Ventricular tachycardia
WBC	White blood count

This book is dedicated to all our parents.

1 Cardiac conditions

Basic life support

The aim of basic life support (BLS) is to 'buy time' until action may be taken to reverse the underlying cause of cardiorespiratory arrest. Chest compressions and artificial ventilation slow the deterioration of the brain, prolong the time period available for successful resuscitation and increase the chance of survival.

The SAFE approach

- Shout for help.
- Approach with care – be aware of potential risks in the immediate environment (e.g. traffic, gas, water) and try to minimise them.
- Free from danger – ensure that the situation is safe before you treat a casualty. Reduce the risk of infection transmission by using gloves and eye protection if at all possible. Also consider the use of a face mask with a one-way valve if this is available.
- Evaluate ABC (airway, breathing and circulation).

Check consciousness

- Check the casualty's response.
  - Ask a question (e.g. 'Are you all right?').
  - Gently shake their shoulders.
- If the casualty is responsive, leave them in the same position (if it is safe to do so), check their condition and call for help if necessary. Reassess them regularly.
- If there is no response, call for help.

Airway

- Open the airway.
  - Place your hand on the casualty's forehead and tilt their head back.
  - Remove any visible obstruction from the mouth (leaving well-fitting dentures *in situ*).
  - Place your fingertips under the point of the casualty's chin and gently lift.
- All injuries that occur at or above the clavicle should be assumed to have resulted in cervical spine trauma until proven otherwise. In these patients, avoid head tilt, and instead use the jaw thrust.
  - Identify the angle of the mandible bilaterally.
  - With all four fingers placed behind each angle of the mandible, steadily push upward and forward to lift the mandible.
  - Use the thumbs to push down gently on the chin to help to open the mouth.

Breathing

- Look, listen and feel for breathing for 10 seconds.
  - Look for chest movements.
  - Listen for breath sounds.
  - Feel for air moving on your cheek.
- If the casualty is breathing normally:
  - place them in the recovery position
  - send for or go to find help.
- If the casualty is not breathing:
  - send for help
  - if you are by yourself, leave the casualty and call for help before beginning cardiopulmonary resuscitation.

Circulation

- Only personnel experienced in clinical assessment should assess the carotid pulse. Lay people should make a diagnosis of cardiac arrest if the victim is unresponsive and not breathing normally.
- If cardiac arrest is diagnosed, begin chest compressions:
  - place the heel of your hand in the centre of the victim's chest
  - place the heel of the other hand on top of this hand, interlock the fingers of both hands and lift them to ensure that pressure is not applied to the ribs

- place yourself vertically above the casualty's chest and press down with straight arms
- depress the sternum by approximately 4–5 cm and then release
- repeat this action at a rate of 100/minute
- even if you hear the ribs break, you should continue basic life support.

Cardiopulmonary resuscitation

- After 30 compressions, reopen the airway and combine compressions with rescue breaths.
- Give two effective rescue breaths.
  - Ensure that the casualty is lying on their back.
  - Ensure that the airway is still open.
  - Pinch the soft part of the nose closed with your thumb and index finger.
  - Take a deep breath and seal your mouth around the casualty's mouth.
  - Blow steadily into the casualty's mouth for 1 second, ensuring that you see the chest rise.
  - Take your mouth away and ensure that the chest wall drops.
  - Repeat the above sequence to deliver a further rescue breath.
  - If there are any problems, recheck the airway.
  - Make up to five attempts to deliver two effective rescue breaths.
- After the two rescue breaths, recommence chest compressions.
- Continue with chest compressions and rescue breaths in a ratio of 30:2.
- Only stop if help arrives, if the casualty shows signs of life or if you become exhausted.

Special circumstances

- In certain situations, the likely cause of unconsciousness will be a breathing problem:
  - drowning
  - children.
- If you are by yourself, perform CPR for 1 minute before going for help.

Further reading

- Resuscitation Council (UK) (2005) *Adult Basic Life Support*. Resuscitation Council (UK), London; www.resus.org.uk/pages/bls.pdf
- Resuscitation Council (UK) and European Resuscitation Council (2004) *Advanced Life Support Manual* (4e revised). Resuscitation Council (UK) and European Resuscitation Council, London.
- St John Ambulance, St Andrew's Ambulance Association and the British Red Cross Society (2002) *First Aid Manual* (8e). Dorling Kindersley Limited, London.

Cardiac arrest: ventricular fibrillation

At the time of cardiac arrest, ventricular fibrillation (VF) is the commonest rhythm seen and has the best prognosis of the cardiac arrest rhythms. VF – and also pulseless ventricular tachycardia (VT) – may be successfully treated by delivering an electrical shock to the heart. It is generally recognised that the shorter the delay before the shock is administered, the better the outcome. It is therefore vitally important that the cardiac rhythm is determined as quickly as possible.

However, recent evidence has found that a period of cardiopulmonary resuscitation (CPR) prior to defibrillation may improve survival in prolonged collapse. Therefore, health professionals attending an unwitnessed cardiac arrest outside of hospital should give CPR for 2 minutes before attempting defibrillation.

Praecordial thump

If an arrest is witnessed by a healthcare professional, a praecordial thump should be administered immediately. This sharp blow with a closed fist over the patient's sternum may convert the patient's cardiac rhythm back to a perfusing rhythm.

Defibrillation

- Apply gel pads and defibrillator paddles (or adhesive electrodes if using an automated external defibrillator) to the patient's chest, one below the right clavicle and the other over the cardiac apex.
- Assess the rhythm (+/–) and check the pulse.
- If VF or pulseless VT is identified:
    - give a single 200J shock
    - recommence CPR for 2 minutes.

Cardiopulmonary resuscitation

CPR should be administered using a ratio of 30 compressions to 2 ventilations. During this time:

- consider and correct any reversible causes of cardiac arrest (see below)
- check the electrode/paddle position
- attempt to secure the airway by means of tracheal intubation/ laryngeal mask airway
- establish intravenous access.

Further defibrillation

- After 2 minutes of CPR, reassess the rhythm.
- If VF/pulseless VT persist, give a further single shock of 360J followed immediately by 2 minutes of CPR.
- Continue loops of 2 minutes of CPR and a single shock of 360J while the patient remains in pulseless VT/VF.
- If VF/pulseless VT persist after 2 shocks, give epinephrine. The dose should be administered before the third shock and repeated before alternate shocks (approximately every 3–5 minutes) – its α-adrenergic actions cause vasoconstriction, improving myocardial and cerebral perfusion pressures and thereby increasing the efficacy of CPR (1 mg IV or 2–3 mg diluted in 10 ml sterile water via the tracheal route).
- Consider drugs for refractory VF.
- If the rhythm changes, check for a pulse:
  - follow the appropriate algorithm if the patient is still pulseless.

Potentially reversible causes

Consider, identify and treat the 4 H's and 4 T's:

- hypoxia
- hypovolaemia
- hypo/hyperkalaemia and other metabolic disorders
- hypothermia
- tension pneumothorax
- tamponade (cardiac)
- toxic/therapeutic disorders
- thrombo-embolic and mechanical obstruction.

Drug treatment for refractory VF

Once epinephrine has been administered, other drug treatments may be considered for shock-resistant VF.

- Amiodarone 300 mg IV may be given before the fourth shock. A further dose of 150 mg may be given for recurrent or refractory VF/pulseless VT.
- Magnesium (4 ml of 50% magnesium sulphate) should be given if there is any suspicion of hypomagnesaemia (e.g. patients on potassium-losing diuretics).
- Lidocaine may be used as an alternative if there is no amiodarone available.

- Consider the use of bicarbonate (50 mmol) if the cardiac arrest is secondary to hyperkalaemia (e.g. renal failure) or a tricyclic overdose. It may also be used if the arterial pH is less than 7.1.

Further reading

- Resuscitation Council (UK) (2005) *Adult Advanced Life Support*. Resuscitation Council (UK), London; www.resus.org.uk/pages/als.pdf
- Resuscitation Council (UK) and European Resuscitation Council (2004) *Advanced Life Support Manual* (4e revised). Resuscitation Council (UK) and European Resuscitation Council, London.
- Rosenberg M, Wang C, Hoffman-Wilde S and Hickham D (1993) Results of cardiopulmonary resuscitation. *Arch Intern Med.* **153:** 1370–5.

Cardiac arrest: pulseless electrical activity

Pulseless electrical activity (PEA), also known as electromechanical dissociation, may be diagnosed when a patient shows signs of a cardiac arrest, but the ECG pattern is compatible with a cardiac output.

Management

- Check the airway.
- Begin cardiopulmonary resuscitation (CPR) with a ratio of 30 compressions to every 2 ventilations.
- Check the electrode/paddle position.
- Attempt to secure the airway by means of tracheal intubation/laryngeal mask airway.
- Establish intravenous access.
- Give epinephrine every 3–5 minutes.
- If the ECG pattern in PEA shows a pulse of less than 60 beats/minute (i.e. a bradycardia), atropine should be administered (3 mg IV or 6 mg via a tracheal tube).
- Reassess the rhythm after 2 minutes:
  - if there is no change in the ECG appearance, continue CPR
  - if the ECG changes and organised electrical activity is seen, check for a pulse.

Potentially reversible causes

The key to successful management of PEA is to identify and treat the underlying cause. Consider the 4 H's and 4 T's.

- Hypoxia – ensure that there is adequate ventilation. Is the chest wall rising? Are there bilateral breath sounds? Is the airway secure with the tracheal tube in the correct position?
- Hypovolaemia:
  - this usually results from severe haemorrhage (e.g. following trauma or a ruptured aortic aneurysm)
  - pregnant women may show signs of hypovolaemia if the pregnant uterus lies over and occludes the inferior vena cava or aorta. This may be avoided by placing a wedge beneath the woman's right hip and manually moving the uterus to the left.

- Hypo/hyperkalaemia and other metabolic disorders:
  - this cause may be suggested by the patient's history (e.g. hyperkalaemia in a patient with renal failure, or hypermagnesaemia in a woman treated for pre-eclampsia)
  - an ECG may be diagnostic, or the condition may be diagnosed by blood tests.
- Hypothermia:
  - this should be considered in all patients who have had a near-drowning experience
  - it should also be considered in patients who have had a prolonged resuscitative attempt.
- Tension pneumothorax:
  - this condition is more common in asthmatics and following major trauma
  - it may also be caused iatrogenically following central line insertion
  - the diagnosis should be made clinically – on the basis of decreased air entry and a hyper-resonant percussion note on the affected side, with tracheal deviation away from the site of pneumothorax
  - the pneumothorax should be decompressed by insertion of a large bore cannula into the second intercostal space over the mid-clavicular line. A chest drain should then be sited. Do not defer decompression to wait for a chest X-ray.
- Tamponade (cardiac):
  - this tends to occur after penetrating chest trauma (and following cardiac surgery)
  - it may be difficult to diagnose at the time of arrest, as the cardinal signs (hypotension, muffled heart sounds and distended neck veins) will all be absent
  - if suspected, attempt needle pericardiocentesis (further details are given in the section on cardiac tamponade; *see* p. 30).
- Toxic/therapeutic disorders:
  - this is an uncommon cause of cardiac arrest, but may be suggested by the history or by the results of biochemical tests
  - it is particularly important to protect the airway in these patients, as there is a high risk of aspiration of stomach contents.
- Thrombo-embolic and mechanical obstruction:
  - the commonest cause is massive pulmonary embolus
  - treatment options include thrombolysis and operative removal of the thrombus (thrombectomy).

Further reading

- Resuscitation Council (UK) (2005) *Adult Advanced Life Support*. Resuscitation Council (UK), London; www.resus.org.uk/pages/als. pdf
- Resuscitation Council (UK) and European Resuscitation Council (2004) *Advanced Life Support Manual* (4e revised). Resuscitation Council (UK) and European Resuscitation Council, London.

Cardiac arrest: asystole

Diagnosis

- Asystole should only be confirmed after:
    - checking that the monitoring leads are firmly and correctly attached
    - checking that the gain is increased
    - checking the rhythm in both leads I and II.
- It is important that this rhythm is not confused with fine ventricular fibrillation (VF).
- In addition, the rhythm should be carefully observed for any evidence of P-wave or slow ventricular activity, since these may benefit from cardiac pacing.

Management

- Check the airway.
- Begin cardiopulmonary resuscitation with a ratio of 30 compressions to 2 ventilations.
- Check the electrode/paddle position.
- Attempt to secure the airway by means of tracheal intubation/laryngeal mask airway.
- Establish intravenous access.
- Give epinephrine every 3–5 minutes.
- Give a single dose of atropine to block the vagus nerve (either 3 mg intravenously or 6 mg via tracheal tube).
- Recheck the rhythm after 2 minutes.
- If asystole persists continue CPR.
- Consider and correct any potentially reversible causes.

Prognosis

Asystole has the poorest prognosis of the cardiac arrest rhythms. It is highly unlikely that successful resuscitation will be achieved after 20 minutes of continuous asystole, despite CPR (unless there is a reversible cause, such as hypothermia).

Further reading

- Resuscitation Council (UK) (2005) *Adult Advanced Life Support.* Resuscitation Council (UK), London; www.resus.org.uk/pages/als.pdf
- Resuscitation Council (UK) and European Resuscitation Council (2004) *Advanced Life Support Manual* (4e revised). Resuscitation Council (UK) and European Resuscitation Council, London.
- VanHoeyweghen R, Mullie A and Bossaert L (1989) Decision making to cease or to continue cardiopulmonary resuscitation. *Resuscitation.* **17:** 137–47.

Acute coronary syndrome

Acute coronary syndrome (ACS) is a term used to describe the processes of unstable angina (myocardial ischaemia at rest) or myocardial infarction. It is usually manifested as a result of thrombus formation on an atherosclerotic plaque in one of the coronary arteries. Risk factors include smoking, hypertension, diabetes mellitus, hypercholesterolaemia and family history of ischaemic heart disease.

Clinical features

The patient may have any or all of the following symptoms:

- chest pain, which is tight or heavy, central and radiates to the jaw and/or arms
- shortness of breath
- nausea or vomiting.

In addition, there may be signs of the following:

- heart failure – pulmonary or ankle oedema, raised jugulovenous pressure (JVP)
- cardiogenic shock (only in massive MI) – hypotension, cold peripheries.

Initial assessment of the patient with 'cardiac' chest pain

Anyone with persistent (duration > 15 minutes) 'cardiac'-sounding chest pain despite the administration of sublingual glyceryl trinitrate (GTN) should be managed as if they have ACS. This includes the following:

- administration of high-flow oxygen via a mask
- ECG
- chest X-ray to look for evidence of pulmonary oedema
- aspirin 300 mg given immediately.

See Figure 1 for an overview of the further management of ACS.

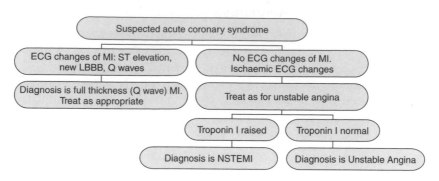

Figure 1 Overview of management of acute coronary syndrome

Management of unstable angina/
non-ST-elevation MI (NSTEMI)

If the ECG demonstrates ischaemia (ST depression or T-wave inversion):

- Commence IV GTN infusion (50 mg in 50 ml normal saline), increasing the rate gradually from 0.5 to 10 mg per hour until the patient is pain-free or the systolic blood pressure drops below 90 mmHg.
- Use subcutaneous low-molecular-weight heparin (e.g. enoxaparin 1 mg/kg twice daily) until the patient has been pain-free for 48 hours.
- Give a β-blocker such as atenolol or metoprolol in order to decrease the demands on the heart. Do not use such drugs if there is severe left ventricular impairment.
- Start an ACE inhibitor such as lisinopril, especially in the presence of left ventricular failure or diabetes mellitus.
- Blood samples for troponin I measurement should be taken. A raised troponin level indicates that a non-ST-elevation myocardial infarction (NSTEMI) has occurred. Clopidogrel 75 mg daily should therefore be given for one year. A normal troponin level confirms the presence of unstable angina.
- Blood samples for measurement of serum lipids should also be taken, and a statin should be commenced if appropriate.
- Senior help is needed if the chest pain does not subside or the ECG changes become more marked, as the patient is at high risk of MI. Where facilities are available, the patient should be referred for acute coronary angioplasty.

Management of full-thickness (Q-wave) MI

In a full-thickness (Q-wave) MI, the ECG demonstrates changes such as ST elevation (at least 2 mm in two adjacent chest leads or at least 1 mm in two adjacent limb leads), new Q-waves or new left bundle branch block. Initially, IV morphine should be given immediately for pain relief. Coronary reperfusion must be re-attempted as soon as possible. Acute angioplasty has been shown to be the most effective mode of coronary reperfusion, although the commonest modality employed in the UK is thrombolysis.

Thrombolysis

Thrombolysis causes plasmin-mediated breakdown of thrombin to dissolve the thrombus. It is most effective if given within 12 hours of the onset of symptoms, and should be performed in a coronary care unit.

The risks of thrombolysis must be explained to the patient. They include the following:

- 1% chance of cerebral haemorrhage
- hypotension
- arrhythmias (therefore the patient must undergo cardiac monitoring).

Absolute contraindications include the following:

- major surgery within the last month
- any past history of cerebral haemorrhage
- uncontrolled hypertension.

Relative contraindications include the following:

- pregnancy
- proliferative diabetic retinopathy
- recent trauma.

Choice of thrombolytic agent

Streptokinase (1.5 million units over 1 hour) is the most commonly used thrombolytic agent. However, recombinant tissue plasminogen activator (rTPA) is used instead of streptokinase if:

- streptokinase has been used before (as antibodies to the drug develop)
- the patient is a young man (< 50 years) with evidence of a large anterior MI, since there is evidence that rTPA results in a lower mortality in these patients.

Other treatments for MI

In addition to reperfusion, the following should be commenced:

- aspirin 75 mg daily
- clopidogrel 75 mg daily for 1 year
- a β-blocker unless severe left ventricular failure is present
- an ACE inhibitor
- a statin (if appropriate).

The use of a GpIIb/IIIa receptor antagonist such as tirofiban may be considered as an adjunct to thrombolysis, since it may improve coronary artery patency and reduce re-occlusion.

Further reading

- Gershlick AH and More RS (1998) Recent advances: treatment of myocardial infarction. *BMJ*. **316**: 280–4.
- Antman EM, Giugliano RP, Gibson CM *et al.* (1999) Abciximab facilitates the rate and extent of thrombolysis: results of the Thrombolysis in Myocardial Infarction (TIMI) 14 trial. *Circulation*. **99**: 2720–32.
- Yusuf S, Mehta SR, Zhao F *et al.* (2003) Early and late effects of clopidogrel in patients with acute coronary syndromes. *Circulation*. **107**: 966.

Narrow complex tachycardia

A narrow complex tachycardia indicates the presence of a supraventricular tachycardia (SVT). However, SVT can appear as a broad
complex tachycardia if it is associated with aberrant conduction (see
below). The different types of SVT include the following:

- atrial fibrillation (AF)
- atrial flutter
- atrioventricular (AV) re-entry tachycardia
- AV nodal re-entry tachycardia.

Clinical features of SVT

These are identical to those of broad complex tachycardia (*see* p. 20).

Management of SVT

See Figure 2 for a summary of management.

- Establish IV access and give oxygen.
- If the rhythm is AF, follow the AF protocol described below.
- Attempt to terminate the SVT with a manoeuvre to increase vagal
  tone. Two such methods are described below.
  - Valsalva manoeuvre – get the patient to blow into a 20-ml syringe
    and try to push the plunger out.
  - Carotid sinus massage – gently massage the carotid at the location
    of its pulse. Do not attempt this if there is a carotid bruit, otherwise
    this may lead to embolism of an atheromatous plaque!
- If vagal manoeuvres are unsuccessful, give IV adenosine. This causes
  short-term (a few seconds) AV block and will terminate some SVTs,
  particularly atrial flutter. It also transiently slows down the tachycardia, enabling recognition of AF. Adenosine must be given with
  cardiac monitoring. Initially try 6 mg adenosine IV. If this is unsuccessful, give 12 mg and then 18 mg. Warn the patient that they may
  experience transient chest tightness and nausea. *Do not give adenosine
  to individuals who suffer from angina, asthma or Wolff–Parkinson–
  White syndrome.*
- If adenosine does not terminate the tachycardia, call for senior help.
  Further treatment depends on the presence of adverse features such as
  a systolic blood pressure of less than 90 mmHg, chest pain, heart
  failure, or a heart rate of more than 200 beats/minute.

  – If adverse factors are present, DC cardioversion is indicated.
  – If no adverse factors are present, anti-arrhythmic drugs such as digoxin, a β-blocker, verapamil or amiodarone may be tried.

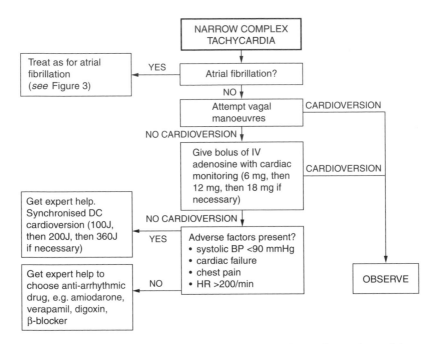

Figure 2   Management of narrow complex tachycardia. Adapted from Resuscitation Council UK (2001)

Management of atrial fibrillation

See Figure 3 for a summary of management.

● Give oxygen, establish IV access and perform cardiac monitoring.
● If the patient is haemodynamically unstable, DC cardioversion or IV amiodarone must be given in order to effect rapid cardioversion.
● If the patient is haemodynamically stable, but is breathless or has a heart rate of less than 100 beats/minute, you must decide which immediate strategy to employ, based on the likely duration of the AF.
  – If the duration of AF is more than 24 hours, there is a high risk of atrial thrombus formation, so do not attempt cardioversion until the patient has been on warfarin for 4 weeks. Treat the AF with rate control via digoxin. A β-blocker, verapamil or diltiazem may

be used for rate control if the patient has good left ventricular function.

– If the duration of AF is less than 24 hours, there is a low risk of atrial thrombus formation, and you should therefore aim for acute cardioversion. Discuss with senior colleagues whether heparinisation followed by IV flecainide, IV amiodarone or DC cardioversion should be attempted.

● If the patient is asymptomatic or has a heart rate of less than 100 beats per minute, no immediate treatment is needed. They will require warfarinisation followed by non-urgent cardioversion if indicated.

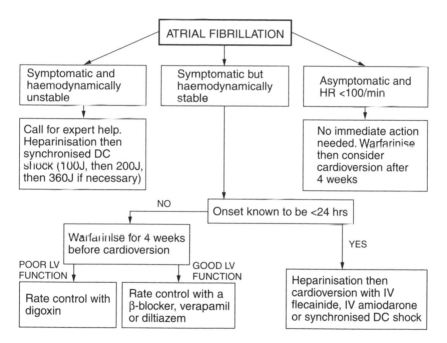

Figure 3 Management of atrial fibrillation. Adapted from Resuscitation Council UK (2001)

Further reading

● Resuscitation Council UK (2001) *Peri-Arrest Arrhythmias*. Resuscitation Council UK, London; www.resus.org.uk/pages/periarst.htm

Broad complex tachycardia

A broad complex tachycardia represents either a ventricular tachycardia (VT) or a supraventricular tachycardia (SVT) with aberrant conduction (e.g. left or right bundle branch block). Close inspection of the ECG may reveal the origin of the tachycardia. The following all suggest a ventricular origin:

● fusion beats
● capture beats
● concordance – the direction of QRS is the same in all leads
● extreme axis deviation.

However, if there is any doubt as to whether the rhythm is VT or SVT, you should assume that the rhythm is VT.

Clinical features

These include the following:

● cardiac failure – raised JVP, pulmonary oedema, peripheral oedema
● hypotension
● cold peripheries
● clammy skin
● pallor
● drowsiness, coma
● oliguria or anuria.

Management of ventricular tachycardia

See Figure 4 for a summary of management.

● If the broad complex tachycardia is believed to be due to SVT then treat as for narrow complex tachycardia, but if in doubt treat as for VT.
● Obtain IV access, give oxygen and use cardiac monitoring.
● Check the serum potassium levels and give IV supplementation if they are below 4.0 mM.
● Check the serum magnesium levels and give 10–20 mM intravenously if needed.
● *Any* tachycardia must be treated immediately with DC cardioversion if the patient has chest pain, acute cardiac failure or hypotension.

● If the patient is stable, attempt chemical cardioversion with amiodarone (150 mg IV over 10 minutes) or lignocaine (lidocaine, 50 mg IV over 2 minutes, which may be repeated every 5 minutes up to a maximum dose of 200 mg). *Note:* Amiodarone should be given centrally to prevent thrombophlebitis.

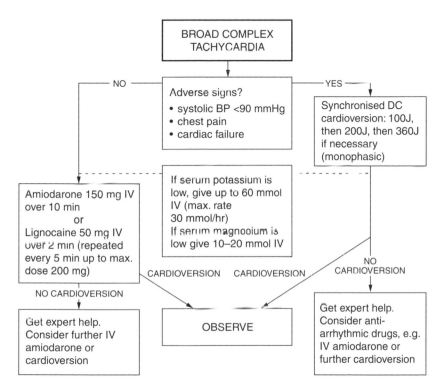

Figure 4   Management of broad complex tachycardia. Adapted from Resuscitation Council UK (2001)

Further reading

● Resuscitation Council UK (2001) *Peri-Arrest Arrhythmias.* Resuscitation Council UK, London; www.resus.org.uk/pages/periarst.htm

Bradycardia

Bradycardia is an abnormally low heart rate (< 60 beats/minute). It commonly occurs physiologically in fit individuals such as athletes. However, inappropriate bradycardia for the haemodynamic state of the patient may cause cardiac failure and require urgent treatment. *See* Table 1 for a classification of bradycardia.

Table 1   Classification of bradycardia

Category of bradycardia	*Examples*
Sinus bradycardia	Physiological (e.g. in athletes)
	Hypothyroidism
	Hypothermia
	Inferior myocardial infarction
	Sick sinus syndrome (degenerative disease of the sino-atrial node)
Heart block	First degree – prolonged PR (> 0.2 seconds)
	Second degree:
	● Mobitz type I (progressively increasing PR)
	● Mobitz type II (2:1, 3:1 or 4:1 AV block)
	Third degree (complete AV dissociation)
Drugs	β-blockers
	Digoxin toxicity
	Amiodarone toxicity

Clinical features

Affected individuals may complain of lethargy, near syncope, syncope or angina. Clinically the patient may show signs of acute left-sided cardiac failure:

● hypotension (systolic blood pressure < 90 mmHg)
● shock
● confusion, drowsiness or coma due to cerebral hypoperfusion
● oliguria/anuria.

Management

See Figure 5 for a summary of management.

- First, decide whether the patient appears to be compromised by the bradycardia in any way. Therefore look for hypotension, shock, or evidence of cerebral or renal hypoperfusion. If any of these are present, give 500 mcg atropine IV.
- If there is no response to the initial dose of atropine, give further 500 mcg doses of atropine up to a total of 3 mg.
- If the patient remains haemodynamically compromised after the maximal dose of atropine, they will need temporary transvenous pacing. Contact the on-call medical or cardiology registrar to arrange this.
- In addition, even if the patient does not appear to be compromised by the bradycardia (with or without atropine), look for the following adverse factors:
  - third-degree heart block with broad QRS complex
  - Mobitz type II heart block
  - ventricular pauses > 3 seconds
  - recent asystole

If any of these adverse factors are present, the patient should be referred for temporary pacing in any case, due to the high risk of asystolic arrest.

- Until temporary transvenous pacing can be performed, transcutaneous pacing or an adrenaline infusion (2–10 mcg/minute) may be used to maintain cardiac output as an interim measure.

Further reading

- Resuscitation Council UK (2001) *Peri-Arrest Arrhythmias*. Resuscitation Council UK, London; www.resus.org.uk/pages/periarst.htm

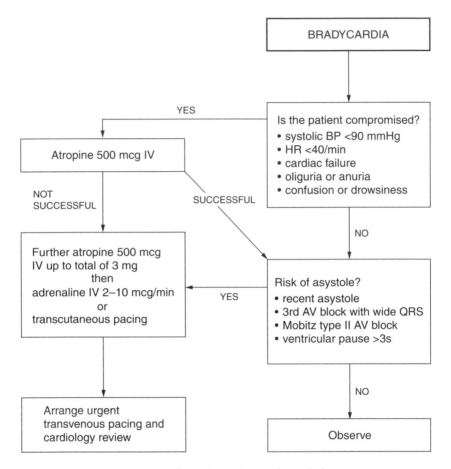

Figure 5 Management of bradycardia. Adapted from Resuscitation Council UK (2001)

Acute pulmonary oedema

Pulmonary oedema is the accumulation of interstitial fluid in the lungs as a result of back-pressure of blood caused by left-sided cardiac failure. It is therefore a feature of congestive cardiac failure. Acute pulmonary oedema is one of the commonest and most important emergencies for the junior doctor.

Causes of acute pulmonary oedema

These include the following:

- ischaemic heart disease (e.g. acute MI)
- tachyarrhythmia (e.g. fast AF)
- bradyarrhythmia (e.g. complete heart block)
- valvular heart disease (e.g. acute mitral incompetence from an MI)
- high-output failure (e.g. severe anaemia, thyrotoxicosis)
- acute renal failure causing oliguria or anuria
- excessive IV fluids.

Clinical features

Features of both left- and right-sided failure are often present in congestive cardiac failure.

Features of left-sided failure

These include the following:

- tachycardia
- third heart sound
- pulmonary oedema – coarse bilateral crackles sparing the apices
- bilateral pleural effusions
- hypotension.

Features of right-sided failure

These include the following:

- raised JVP
- pitting oedema in the legs, extending proximally.

Management

- Sit the patient up! This step reduces the pulmonary oedema, and therefore immediately helps breathing.
- Administer high-flow oxygen (15 litres/minute) via a mask with a re-breathe bag.
- Stop all IV fluids, as they will worsen fluid overload.
- Give IV furosemide 40 mg immediately.
- Make sure that the patient is catheterised so that any diuresis may be measured.
- Get an urgent, portable chest radiograph to confirm the diagnosis. Look for pulmonary oedema, upper lobe diversion, Kerley B lines and pleural effusions.
- Measure arterial blood gases.
- Morphine 5 mg IM is a useful anxiolytic agent and vasodilator.
- If the patient is very breathless, commence a glyceryl trinitrate (GTN) infusion (50 mg in 50 ml of normal saline) to reduce pre-load via vasodilatation. Start at 0.5 mg per hour, and increase the rate gradually to a maximum of 10 mg per hour, or until the patient's blood pressure drops to 90 mmHg.
- Perform an ECG to rule out an arrhythmia such as fast AF. Look for ECG signs of pulmonary embolism, including sinus tachycardia (most common), new right bundle branch block and S1 Q3 T3 (unusual).
- Check the following:
  - FBC – is the patient anaemic?
  - U&Es – acute renal impairment may cause pulmonary oedema
  - thyroid function tests – but beware of sick euthyroid syndrome
  - troponin I – 12 hours after the onset of symptoms.
- Withhold any β-blockers, since they will worsen acute cardiac failure (although they are beneficial in chronic cardiac failure).
- If adequate diuresis (at least 500 ml within the first hour) does not occur, give further doses of IV furosemide.
- If rapid clinical improvement does not occur, call senior colleagues for help. Further therapy includes continuous positive airways pressure (CPAP), or even invasive ventilation.

Malignant hypertension

Malignant (accelerated) hypertension is defined as hypertension associated with rapid, progressive end-organ damage such as retinopathy, encephalopathy or renal failure. If it is left untreated, further complications such as aortic dissection and cerebral infarction may occur.

Aetiology

Malignant hypertension is a rare complication of any cause of hypertension. Around 95% of cases of hypertension are primary/idiopathic. Major causes of secondary hypertension are listed in Table 2.

Table 2   Classification of secondary hypertension

Category	Cause of hypertension
Renal	Acute renal failure Renal artery stenosis Polycystic kidney disease
Cardiac	Coarction of aorta
Endocrine	Phaeochromocytoma Conn's syndrome Cushing's syndrome Congenital adrenal hyperplasia
Pregnancy	Pre-eclampsia
Drugs	Steroids Sympathomimetics (e.g. cocaine, amphetamines)

Clinical features

Look for evidence of acute end-organ damage. This includes the following:

- retinopathy – grade 3 or 4 hypertensive retinopathy may be seen on fundoscopy (*see* Table 3)
- acute renal failure – signs of fluid overload such as peripheral oedema, pulmonary oedema and raised JVP may be present
- encephalopathy – confusion, agitation, drowsiness or even coma may be present.

There may also be evidence of acute cardiac failure.

Table 3   Classification of hypertensive retinopathy

Grade of retinopathy	Features seen on fundoscopy
1	'Silver-wiring' – increased reflective capacity of arteries
2	Arteriovenous nipping
3	Grade 2 retinopathy + cotton-wool spots and flame-shaped or blot haemorrhages
4	Grade 3 retinopathy + papilloedema

Management

It is extremely important not to try to reduce blood pressure too abruptly, as this may lead to watershed cerebral infarction.

- Ideally the patient should be monitored in a high-dependency unit.
- Perform an ECG to look for evidence of long-standing hypertension (i.e. left ventricular hypertrophy).
- Check urinalysis for proteinuria and send blood for U&Es, to check for evidence of renal failure.
- Perform fundoscopy to look for evidence of hypertensive retinopathy.
- Aim to reduce the diastolic blood pressure to 100 mmHg, or by 15–20 mmHg in the first 24 hours.
- If there is only mild evidence of end-organ involvement, try an oral agent such as amlodipine. However, if there is more advanced end-organ damage, discuss the choice of drug treatment with senior colleagues. Options include the following:
  - IV labetolol
  - IV hydralazine
  - IV sodium nitroprusside (note that this infusion needs to be wrapped in silver foil to prevent degradation in ambient light).
- Once the blood pressure is under control, an oral antihypertensive agent may be prescribed regularly.
- It is always important to investigate the patient for causes of secondary hypertension.

Further reading

- Elliot WJ (2004) Clinical features and management of selected hypertensive emergencies. *Clin Hypertens.* **6**: 587–92.

Cardiac tamponade

Causes

Cardiac tamponade describes the state of compromised cardiac output due to the accumulation of fluid (usually blood) within the pericardial sac. This commonly results from penetrating thoracic trauma, but infrequently can also be due to blunt injury to the heart, great vessels or pericardial vessels. Because the pericardial sac is a fixed, fibrous structure, it only takes a relatively small amount of blood (20 ml or so) to restrict the pumping action of the heart and therefore decrease stroke volume, leading to a diminished cardiac output (remember that cardiac output = stroke volume × heart rate). Cardiac tamponade is also a post-operative complication of cardiac surgery, especially if the pericardium is opened. Furthermore, to allow surgery on a still heart the circulation must be temporarily replaced with a cardiopulmonary bypass machine to take over the pumping and oxygenation of blood. As blood passes through the bypass circuit, platelets are consumed (hence cardiac surgery and bypass are causes of disseminated intravascular coagulation), further increasing the risk of haemorrhage into the pericardiac sac.

Diagnosis

The effects of tamponade to the heart are those of an obstructive shock picture, namely a rise in venous pressure and a decline in arterial pressure. Because blood is occupying the space between the heart and the doctor's stethoscope, the heart sounds are distant and muffled. These three signs (raised JVP, decreased blood pressure and muffled heart sounds) form the classic Beck's triad that is diagnostic of cardiac tamponade. In addition, due to the presence of blood in the pericardium, the cardiac shadow appears enlarged on chest X-ray. Pulsus paradoxus is a normal physiological decrease in systolic blood pressure that occurs during inspiration, but when exaggerated this is another sign of cardiac tamponade. Kussmaul's sign describes the rise in venous pressure (manifested clinically by the JVP) during inspiration (venous pressure normally *falls* during inspiration).

Cardiac tamponade is the commonest cause of PEA (also known as electromechanical dissociation; *see* p. 8) in the absence of tension pneumothorax and hypovolaemia.

In the emergency setting it can be difficult to assess the audibility of heart sounds, and trauma patients may be hypovolaemic, which results in a lowering of the patient's blood pressure and JVP. Consequently, cardiac tamponade rarely presents with the full Beck's triad. Pulsus paradoxus and Kussmaul's sign are often subtle, and PEA has numerous causes. For these reasons it is vital to maintain a high index of suspicion for the diagnosis of cardiac tamponade. Transthoracic echocardiography (TTE) is not considered sensitive enough for diagnosis, and ultrasound examination of the pericardial sac is not a skill in which most UK surgeons have sufficient competence. The trauma team should therefore proceed directly to evacuation of pericardial blood in any patient who does not respond to the usual resuscitation measures for haemorrhagic shock (*see* Chapter 11, section on circulation; p. 156), and who has the potential for cardiac tamponade.

Management

First, evaluate ABC (*see* Chapter 11, section on general principles; p. 149). Cardiac tamponade is dealt with under 'C' (although it can also be regarded as a 'B' cause because of its effects on ventilation).

The easiest and quickest way to evacuate pericardial blood in the trauma patient is by a subxiphoid pericardiocentesis. If the cardiac surgeon is present at the trauma call/ cardiac arrest, he or she may prefer to perform a subxiphoid pericardiac window or emergency thoracotomy and pericardiotomy instead, especially if the blood has clotted. In the case of post-operative patients, cardiac surgeons often prefer to take the patient back to theatre, so medical students and junior doctors are best advised to call them rather than to institute management themselves. However, pericardiocentesis is one of the few simple truly life-saving manoeuvres, and all emergency medical staff should be competent in this procedure.

During preparation for pericardiocentesis, fluid resuscitation according to ABC principles will improve the venous pressure and cardiac output. A large-bore needle with a syringe on its end is inserted just below the xiphoid process in the direction of the left shoulder tip (remember that the tip of the shoulder is at the inferior aspect of the shoulder blade). An ECG monitor should be connected to check that the needle is not inserted into the heart itself (indicated by needle-induced dysrhythmias). After positive pericardiocentesis following trauma, the patient should be referred to a cardiac surgeon for inspection of the heart via open thoracotomy or median sternotomy.

Further reading

- American College of Surgeons Committee on Trauma (2004) *Advanced Trauma Life Support for Doctors: student course manual* (7e). American College of Surgeons Committee on Trauma, Chicago.
- Ellis H, Calne R and Watson C (1998) *Lecture Notes in General Surgery* (9e). Blackwell Science, Oxford.

2 Respiratory conditions

Acute asthma

Acute asthma is a common condition, with approximately 5.2 million sufferers in the UK. There are approximately 1400 deaths attributed to asthma every year, a third of these occurring in people under the age of 65 years. These deaths are potentially avoidable, as acute asthma is a largely reversible condition. The majority of deaths occur in the community and in patients with chronically severe asthma, often due to inadequate steroid treatment, inadequate objective measures of asthma and poor follow-up.

Clinical features

These are summarised in Tables 4 and 5.

Table 4 Clinical features of acute asthma in adults

Moderate	Severe	Life-threatening
PEF 50–75% of best or predicted rate Increasing symptoms No features of severe asthma	Any one of: • PEF 33–50% of best or predicted rate • RR ≥ 25 breaths/min • Pulse ≥ 110 beats/min • Cannot complete full sentences in one breath	Any one of: • PEF < 33% of best or predicted rate • $SaO_2 < 92\%$ • Silent chest • Feeble respiratory effort • Cyanosis • Bradycardia, hypotension or dysrhythmia • Confusion • Exhaustion • Coma

PEF, peak expiratory flow; RR, respiratory rate.

Table 5   Clinical features of acute asthma in children

Acute severe	Life-threatening

Cannot complete sentences in one breath, or too breathless to talk or feed
Pulse: > 120 beats/min in children > 5 years
        > 130 beats/min in children aged 2–5 years
RR: > 30 breaths/min in children > 5 years
        > 50 breaths/min in children aged 2–5 years
PEF < 50% of best or predicted rate
	PEF < 33% of best or predicted rate
	Silent chest
	Poor respiratory effort
	Cyanosis
	Hypotension
	Confusion
	Reduced level of consciousness
	Coma

Management

Moderate exacerbation in adults

- Administer oxygen.
- Give salbutamol or terbutaline – 4–6 puffs via large-volume spacer or nebuliser.
- Monitor the patient's response after 15–30 minutes.
- If the symptoms are settling, the patient can be discharged home with management as follows:
  - oral prednisolone 40–50 mg daily for at least 5 days
  - step up the patient's usual treatment
  - ask the patient to monitor symptoms and peak flow, and give them an asthma management plan
  - review within 48 hours.
- Admit the patient to hospital if they show any features of severe or life-threatening asthma or have a history of a previous near-fatal attack.

Severe exacerbation in adults

- Administer oxygen.
- Give salbutamol or terbutaline – oxygen-driven nebuliser or 4–6 puffs via large-volume spacer.
- Give oral prednisolone 40–50 mg or IV hydrocortisone 100 mg.
- Monitor the patient's response after 15–30 minutes.
- If any signs of acute asthma persist, arrange admission. In the meantime, administer repeat nebulised β2 agonist plus ipratropium.

- If symptoms have improved and PEF is > 50% of best or predicted rate, the patient can be discharged home with management as follows:
  - oral prednisolone 40–50 mg daily for at least 5 days
  - step up the patient's usual treatment
  - ask the patient to monitor symptoms and peak flow, and give them an asthma management plan
  - review within 24 hours.

Life-threatening exacerbation in adults

- Arrange immediate hospital admission.
- Administer oxygen.
- Give oxygen-driven nebulised β2 agonist plus ipratropium.
- Give oral prednisolone 40–50 mg or IV hydrocortisone 100 mg.

Hospital care

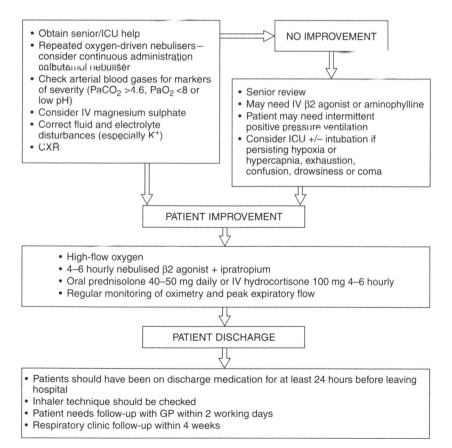

Figure 6   Management of acute asthma

Children

Follow the same principles as above. Treatment can be summarised as follows.

- Salbutamol: age 0–5 years, 2.5 mg nebuliser; age > 5 years, 2.5–5 mg nebuliser.
- Terbutaline: age 0–5 years, 5 mg nebuliser; age > 5 years, 5–10 mg nebuliser.
- Ipratropium: 0.25 mg nebuliser.
- Prednisolone: age < 2 years, 10 mg; age 2–5 years, 20 mg; age > 5 years, 30–40 mg. If already on prednisolone, give 2 mg/kg up to a maximum dose of 60 mg.
- Hydrocortisone: 4 mg/kg.

Further reading

- Scottish Intercollegiate Guideline Network (2004) *Guideline No. 63 British Guideline on the Management of Asthma*; www.sign.ac.uk/guidelines/fulltext/63/index.html

Acute exacerbation of chronic obstructive

pulmonary disease

Chronic obstructive pulmonary disease (COPD) represents the spectrum of lung disease that includes chronic bronchitis and emphysema, and is characterised by chronic, non-reversible airways obstruction. Two classic types of COPD patient exist. Those with predominant emphysema ('blue bloaters') have an impaired respiratory drive, so are cyanosed but hypercapnoeic ($pCO_2 > 6$ kPa). However, patients with predominant chronic bronchitis ('pink puffers') have an intact respiratory drive, so may appear more breathless but are not usually hypercapnoeic.

Causes of exacerbation of COPD

Chest infection is the main cause of exacerbation. Common pathogens include *Haemophilus influenzae*, *Streptococcus pneumoniae* and *Moraxella catarrhalis*. Other causes include the following:

- mucus plugging leading to collapse of a lung lobe or segment
- pneumothorax
- cor pulmonale (right-sided heart failure due to pulmonary hypertension associated with COPD).

Clinical features

Typical symptoms of an exacerbation are increased shortness of breath, wheeze and cough (with purulent sputum). On examination, look for the following signs:

- cyanosis
- tachycardia (> 110 beats/minute)
- tachypnoea (> 30 breaths/minute)
- pursed-lip breathing (which maintains positive airways pressure in expiration in order to minimise airways collapse)
- use of accessory muscles of respiration such as sternocleidomastoids and trapezii
- features of chest hyper-expansion, including intercostal recession, tracheal tug, loss of cardiac and hepatic dullness to percussion
- carbon dioxide retention flap.

Management

- Give 28% oxygen via a Venturi mask (do not give a higher FiO_2 (fraction of inspired oxygen) at this time, since respiratory depression may occur if the patient has chronic carbon dioxide retention – that is, if they are a 'blue bloater').
- Check the arterial blood gases (ABG).
- Nebulised salbutamol 5 mg (every 4 hours) and ipratropium bromide 500 mcg (four times daily) should be given regularly to relieve bronchospasm.
- Monitoring of the peak flow rate (PFR) and comparison of this value with the patient's own best value (ask them!) will indicate the degree of worsening of airways obstruction.
- A chest X-ray is vital to look for pneumothorax, collapse and pneumonia. Other features of COPD may be present, such as hyper-expanded lung fields, flattened diaphragm and bullae.
- Sputum culture and blood cultures should be sent in order to look for evidence of an infective cause.
- A raised white cell count and C-reactive protein (CRP) level indicate infection.
- Antibiotics should be given. Amoxycillin, 500 mg to 1 g (three times daily) administered orally or intravenously, is the first-line agent. In severe cases or if there is no response, use IV cefuroxime, co-amoxyclav or ciprofloxacin.
- Steroids in the form of prednisolone 30 mg daily (or hydrocortisone 100–150 mg daily if the patient cannot swallow) should be given for 1 week.
- If bronchoconstriction does not respond to repeated nebulisers, call for senior colleagues to consider IV aminophylline (loading dose 250 mg over 20 minutes, then administered at a rate of 0.5 mg/kg/ hour adjusted by drug-level monitoring). Cardiac monitoring is essential due to the risk of tachyarrhythmias. Use this treatment with caution if the patient is already on oral theophyllines.

Management of CO_2 retention

This issue often causes anxiety among junior doctors. Oxygen therapy must be guided by two principles:

1 correction of hypoxia ($pO_2 < 8$ kPa) to keep oxygen saturation above 90% (it is unnecessary to aim for higher oxygen saturation levels in these patients)
2 prevention of hypercapnoea ($pCO_2 > 6$ kPa) and drowsiness.

Unfortunately, it is not always possible to correct hypoxia while preventing hypercapnoea. The following steps should therefore be taken when managing these patients (*see* Figure 7).

- If the pCO_2 is < 6 kPa (i.e. the patient is a 'pink puffer'), increase the FiO_2 in order to correct hypoxia until the oxygen saturation is > 90%. Check ABG after 1 hour to ensure that the pCO_2 is still < 6 kPa.
- If the pCO_2 is > 6 kPa (i.e. the patient is a 'blue bloater'), do not give more than 28%, otherwise respiratory depression will occur. The aim is therefore to let the patient remain hypoxic in order to preserve respiratory drive. Monitor ABG every 30 minutes initially in order to check that CO_2 retention is not worsening.
- If worsening CO_2 retention or drowsiness occurs, the FiO_2 must be decreased, and ABG should be monitored after 30 minutes.
- Review by senior colleagues with an assessment of the patient's suitability for bi-level positive-airways-pressure non-invasive ventilation is needed if:
  - the patient remains drowsy or the pCO_2 continues to rise (> 8 kPa) despite a reduction in FiO_2
  - hypoxia is present and a higher FiO_2 cannot be given due to CO_2 retention.

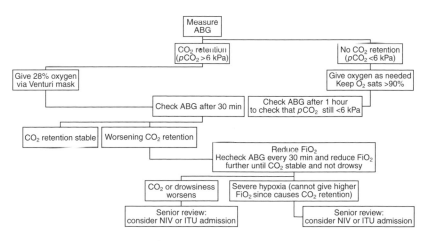

Figure 7   Management of carbon dioxide retention in COPD

Note that respiratory stimulants such as doxepram are no longer recommended, since it is believed that they eventually worsen respiratory fatigue. Consideration of intubation and ventilation in an ITU is needed if bi-level positive airways pressure is not tolerated. However, because of the poor prognosis of some patients with exacerbations of COPD, a decision needs to be made about the appropriateness of such action in each individual case.

Further reading

- National Institute for Clinical Excellence (2004) *Management of Chronic Obstructive Pulmonary Disease in Adults in Primary and Secondary Care*. National Institute for Clinical Excellence, London.
- Hosker H, Cooke NJ and Hawkey P (1994) Antibiotics in chronic obstructive pulmonary disease. *BMJ*. **308:** 871–2.

Pneumothorax

Pneumothorax is defined as air in the pleural space, which is situated between the visceral and parietal layers of the pleura. Tension pneumothorax is a pneumothorax associated with cardiorespiratory compromise. It is caused by the build-up of intrapleural air under high pressure via a valve effect, which leads to displacement of the mediastinum and consequent impairment of cardiac function.

Aetiology of pneumothorax

Primary pneumothorax occurs in previously fit people, classically in tall young men. Secondary pneumothorax occurs in individuals with pre-existing lung disease. Causes of secondary pneumothorax include the following:

- asthma
- chronic obstructive airways disease
- fibrosing alveolitis
- bronchial carcinoma.

Clinical features

The patient may complain of shortness of breath, chest pain or a cough. On examination, the following features may be present:

- tachypnoea
- tachycardia
- tracheal deviation *towards* the pneumothorax
- the following signs are ipsilateral to the pneumothorax:
    - decreased chest expansion
    - decreased breath sounds
    - hyper-resonance on percussion.

However, tension pneumothorax may have the following features:

- rapidly worsening respiratory distress
- hypotension
- raised JVP
- tracheal deviation *away from* the pneumothorax
- deviation of the apex beat *away from* the pneumothorax

- the following signs are ipsilateral to the pneumothorax:
  - decreased chest expansion
  - decreased breath sounds
  - hyper-resonance on percussion.

Management

- Give high-flow oxygen unless the patient is known to have COPD (in which case you should give 28% oxygen).
- Perform a chest radiograph to diagnose the pneumothorax.
- Arterial blood gases should be measured.
- Follow the management plans outlined in Figures 8 and 9.

Management of suspected tension pneumothorax

If you suspect tension pneumothorax in a patient who is in a rapidly deteriorating clinical state with the features described above, you must act immediately.

- Start high-flow oxygen.
- Call for help from senior colleagues.
- *There is no time to get a chest X-ray.* You must therefore act on your clinical findings.
- Insert a large (e.g. brown) venflon into the chest wall anteriorly in the second intercostal space, in the mid-clavicular line. You should hear a hiss of air being forced out of the affected lung, and the patient should immediately improve clinically.
- Now take a chest X-ray and measure ABG. Then insert a chest drain (tube thoracotomy).

Technique for aspiration of a pneumothorax

See Figures 8 and 9 for indications for aspiration of a pneumothorax.

- Using aseptic technique, infiltrate lignocaine (lidocaine, 1% or 2%) into the second intercostal space in the mid-clavicular line.
- Place a large (e.g. brown) venflon attached to a syringe into the second intercostal space until air can be aspirated, and then withdraw the needle.

● Attach a three-way tap and a 50-ml syringe to the cannula.

Aspirate air (expelling it via the three-way tap) until the patient coughs repeatedly, until 2500 ml (the volume of one lung) have been drained or until resistance is felt.

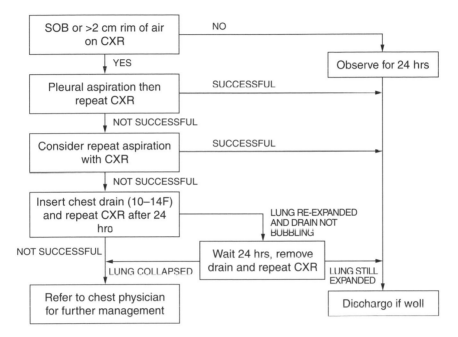

Figure 8   Management of primary pneumothorax

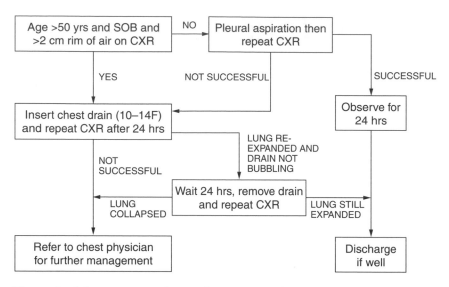

Figure 9   Management of secondary pneumothorax

Further reading

- Henry M, Arnold A and Harvey J on behalf of the British Thoracic Society Pleural Disease Group (2003) The British Thoracic Society guidelines for the management of spontaneous pneumothorax. *Thorax.* 58 (Suppl. II): ii39–52.

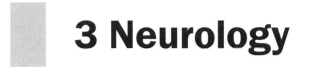

3 Neurology

Coma/reduced consciousness

Reduced consciousness (or coma, in its extreme state) is the brain's common response to any of a multitude of possible causative factors. Most cases should be reversible on treatment of the underlying pathology.

Glasgow Coma Scale

The Glasgow Coma Scale (GCS) is used to quantify the level of consciousness, and must be measured in every patient with reduced consciousness (see Table 6). Every patient will achieve a score of between 15 (completely alert) and 3 (completely comatose).

Table 6   Glasgow Coma Scale

Examined response	Response	Score
Eyes opening	Open spontaneously	4
	Open to verbal command	3
	Open to tactile stimulus	2
	No response (even to pain)	1
Verbal response	Non-confused speech	5
	Confused speech	4
	Incoherent words	3
	Incomprehensible sounds	2
	No response	1
Motor response	Obeys simple commands	6
	Localises to pain	5
	Withdraws from pain	4
	Flexor to pain	3
	Extensor to pain	2
	No movement	1

Aetiology of coma/reduced consciousness

Table 7 lists the different categories of common causes of reduced consciousness.

Table 7 Common causes of reduced consciousness

Category	Causes of reduced consciousness
Neurological	Head injury Seizure or post-ictal state Meningitis/encephalitis Cerebral tumour Hydrocephalus Cerebral haemorrhage
Respiratory	Type 2 respiratory failure
Drugs	Alcohol Benzodiazepines Opioids
Metabolic	Hypoglycaemia Diabetic ketoacidosis Liver failure Renal failure
Cardiac	Shock Arrhythmia
Sepsis	

Management

Before you do anything else, perform the following initial assessments, which will affect subsequent management of the patient.

1 Quickly assess ABC (airway, breathing and circulation) to exclude cardiac arrest.
2 Measure the GCS score. A patient with a GCS score of ≤ 8 cannot protect their own airway, so will need to be placed in the recovery position, given oxygen via a mask, and ventilated using a bag and mask if necessary. The on-call anaesthetist should be called urgently to consider intubation of the patient.

The next step is to look for the underlying cause of coma.

- Check the blood sugar level using glucose stix. Hypoglycaemia is a common and easily reversible cause of coma!
- Hypotension may indicate sepsis (particularly if associated with pyrexia) or other causes of shock.
- Measure the pulse and perform an ECG, looking for evidence of arrhythmia.
- Look at the patient's medical notes.
  - Is there a history of alcoholism?
  - Is there a history of liver or renal failure?
  - Is the patient diabetic?
  - Is there a history of chronic obstructive airways disease?
  - Is there a history of any intracranial pathology (e.g. brain tumour)?
- What drugs is the patient taking? If you suspect opioid overdose (in which case the patient will have pinpoint pupils), give 400 mcg of IV/ IM naloxone. Be warned that the analgesic effects of opioids will be rapidly reversed, which may lead to the patient screaming in pain on recovery.
- Measurement of ABG, looking for evidence of hypoxia, hyper-capnoea or acidosis, is helpful when searching for a respiratory or metabolic cause of coma.
- Perform urinalysis. Is there evidence of a urinary tract infection (UTI)? The presence of ketones in a diabetic patient who is acidotic suggests diabetic ketoacidosis.
- Take a chest X-ray to look for evidence of pneumonia.
- If there is any evidence of sepsis, take cultures and then start empirical antibiotics.
- Perform a full neurological examination.
  - Signs of meningism (e.g. photophobia, neck stiffness) suggest either meningitis or subarachnoid haemorrhage.
  - Is there papilloedema on fundoscopy, which would suggest a raised intracranial pressure (ICP)?
  - Is there evidence of a new focal neurological deficit?

If any of the above features are present, a primary neurological pathology seems likely, and an urgent CT scan of the head is required. If the scan reveals an intracranial mass, haemorrhage or hydrocephalus, the findings must be discussed with the on-call neurosurgical team. If meningitis is suspected, take blood cultures, give empirical antibiotics and perform a lumbar puncture only if the CT scan of the head does *not* demonstrate raised ICP (to prevent coning).

Raised intracranial pressure

Patients with raised intracranial pressure (ICP) normally present with reduced consciousness or coma. Treatment is given to prevent clinical deterioration and herniation of the brainstem through the foramen magnum (coning), which is invariably fatal.

Aetiology

This can be summarised as follows.

- Focal space-occupying lesions:
  - cerebral haemorrhage (subdural, subarachnoid or intracerebral)
  - intracranial tumour
  - intracranial abscess.
- Hydrocephalus (communicating and non-communicating).
- Meningo-encephalitis.
- Head trauma (via cerebral oedema or contusion).
- Benign intracranial hypertension (BIH).

Clinical features

The patient may give a history of throbbing headache that is worse in the morning, nausea and vomiting. On examination, a patient with raised ICP may show:

- reduced consciousness
- papilloedema
- seizures, particularly with focal space-occupying lesions
- false localising signs – displacement of the brain may cause stretching of cranial nerves (particularly the VIth cranial nerve, due to its long intracranial course)
- pyrexia – in the case of cerebral infection
- hypertension and bradycardia (Cushing's reflex) – signs of brainstem compression and imminent coning.

Management

Always request help from senior colleagues when you have a patient with suspected raised ICP.

- Give the patient oxygen via a mask.
- Assess their level of consciousness using the Glasgow Coma Scale (*see* p. 43). If their GCS score is ≤ 8, the patient cannot maintain their airway, so will require endotracheal intubation by the on-call anaesthetist.
- Use glucose stix to rule out the possibility of hypoglycaemia.
- If raised ICP is suspected, perform an urgent CT scan of the brain.
- *Do not* perform a lumbar puncture if there is a focal intracranial lesion or non-communicating hydrocephalus, as this will cause coning and immediate death.
- If possible, tilt the patient to about 30 degrees head-up, in order to promote intracranial venous drainage and thus reduce the ICP.
- Cerebral haemorrhage should be urgently referred for a neuro-surgical opinion.
- Treat patients with suspected meningitis with antibiotics (*see* p. 49). If a cerebral abscess is found, discuss with the microbiologist the choice of antibiotics.
- Intracranial tumours or abscesses typically have a surrounding area of oedema. Dexamethasone (4 mg every 6 hours) reduces the level of oedema and thus the ICP.
- Mannitol (0.5–1 g/kg IV over 20 minutes) is an osmotic diuretic that may be considered in order to relieve raised ICP. However, renal function must be monitored due to the marked diuresis which occurs with this drug.
- Intubation followed by hyperventilation may also be considered in the ITU. This reduces carbon dioxide levels in the blood, thereby promoting vasoconstriction and reducing the movement of fluid into the cerebral tissue.

Meningitis

Meningitis is inflammation of the meninges and cerebrospinal fluid. It is usually caused by a viral infection, but bacterial meningitis is the most deadly form.

Causes of meningitis

Bacterial meningitis

Neisseria meningitidis (meningococcus types A, B and C) is the commonest cause of bacterial meningitis (meningococcal meningitis) in the UK, and is transmitted by respiratory and direct spread. It is also the most dangerous form of meningitis, since septicaemia commonly occurs. The causes of bacterial meningitis are classified according to the age group of the patient (*see* Table 8).

Table 8   Classification of causes of bacterial meningitis by age of patient

Age of patient	Common causes	Less common causes
Neonate	Streptococcus group B	*Listeria monocytogenes*
Infant	*Haemophilus influenzae*	*Neisseria meningitidis* *Streptococcus pneumoniae*
Adult	*Neisseria meningitidis*	*Streptococcus pneumoniae* *Haemophilus influenzae*
Older person	*Streptococcus pneumoniae*	*Neisseria meningitidis*

Other causes of meningitis

These include the following:

- viral causes (these account for 80% of cases of meningitis):
  - enteroviruses such as Coxsackie, polio and ECHO viruses account for most cases
  - influenza
  - mumps
  - herpes simplex, varicella zoster
- immunocompromised patients (e.g. those with HIV, lymphoma, or undergoing chemotherapy):
  - normal pathogens (see above) as well as opportunistic organisms such as TB (may cause chronic meningitis and hydrocephalus)

- fungi (e.g. *Cryptococcus*)
- protozoal infection (e.g. *Toxoplasma*)
- non-infectious meningitis:
  - neoplasms (e.g. lymphoma, metastatic carcinoma such as that of the breast or lung)
  - inflammatory diseases such as systemic lupus erythematosus and sarcoidosis.

Clinical features

Symptoms include fever, meningeal irritation, headache (classically a severe occipital headache), neck stiffness, nausea and vomiting. On examination the following signs may be present:

- high temperature
- reduced consciousness
- purpuric, non-blanching rash – *this only occurs in the meningococcal form (caused by Neisseria meningitidis)*
- neck stiffness, Kernig's sign (with the hip flexed, passive extension at the knee causes spasm in the thigh), Brudzinski's sign (passive flexion of the neck leads to involuntary hip flexion)
- hypotension or shock, especially in the presence of meningococcal septicaemia
- seizures
- false localising signs such as VIth or VIIIth cranial nerve palsies, caused by the stretching of nerve fibres by cerebral oedema
- hydrocephalus (especially in TB meningitis) presenting with increasing drowsiness or coma
- coning – this is lethal herniation of the brainstem through the foramen magnum, caused by cerebral oedema.

Management of bacterial meningitis

It is vital that empirical antibiotics are given immediately if meningitis is suspected. Under no circumstances should any investigation or result delay antibiotic treatment, as bacterial meningitis can progress and worsen over hours, becoming fatal.

- Empirical antibiotic therapy is with high-dose IV cefotaxime (2 g four times daily) or ceftriaxone (2 g twice daily). IV ampicillin (2 g four times daily) should be added in patients over 55 years of age to cover *Listeria* meningitis.

- Rapid IV fluids are given to aggressively treat hypotension or shock (*see* p. 251). If shock has occurred, call for intensive-care assessment.
- Blood cultures should be taken ideally before, but should *never* delay, the administration of any antibiotics. Always take a throat swab.
- A raised white cell/neutrophil count and raised C-reactive protein (CRP) level are consistent with infection. Serial measurement is useful for monitoring the response to therapy. U&Es should be monitored, as sepsis can cause renal failure.
- A CT scan of the head should be performed, as it is important to rule out a focal cerebral lesion such as a subarachnoid haemorrhage before performing a lumbar puncture, otherwise fatal coning may occur.
- A lumbar puncture should be performed and a CSF sample sent for microscopy, culture and biochemical investigations (protein and glucose) (*see* Table 9 for interpretation of CSF analysis). An auramine stain should be performed if TB is suspected. An Indian ink stain will detect *Cryptococcus neoformans* in immunocompromised patients.
- Meningitis is a notifiable disease. Contact tracing is performed by the public health physician once notification has occurred.
- The role of steroids is very controversial. Dexamethasone (0.15 mg/kg four times daily) may have a role if pneumococcal meningitis is suspected.

Table 9   Cerebrospinal fluid analysis for different causes of meningitis and a healthy individual

CSF measurement	Healthy individual	Bacterial meningitis	Viral meningitis	TB meningitis
White cell count	< 5	500–5000 neutrophils	50–1000 lymphocytes	50–5000 lymphocytes
Protein concentration	Up to 0.5 g/litre	High	Normal	High
Glucose concentration	> 2/3 of serum glucose	Low	Normal	Low

Further reading

- Begg N, Cartwright KA, Cohen J et al. (1999) Consensus statement on diagnosis, investigation, treatment and prevention of acute bacterial meningitis in immunocompetent adults. British Infection Society Working Party. *J Infect.* **39**: 1–15.

Stroke

Stroke (also known as cerebrovascular accident) is a syndrome of acute disturbance of cerebral function lasting for more than 24 hours, which is usually caused by thromboembolism in a cerebral artery. Strokes may be preceded by transient ischaemic attacks (TIAs), which cause cerebral deficits that recover fully within 24 hours. A reversible ischaemic neurological deficit (RIND) is similar to a TIA but persists for more than 24 hours.

Aetiology

Most strokes arise from embolism of atherosclerotic material from the carotid arteries or the arch of the aorta. They may also arise from *in-situ* thrombus in the heart, especially in AF or post-MI.

Clinical features

Stroke-related symptoms and signs vary depending on the vascular territory involved (*see* Table 10).

The patient may give a history of predisposing factors such as smoking, hypertension or diabetes. In addition, there may be evidence of AF, a heart murmur or a carotid bruit.

Acute management of stroke

See Figure 10 for a summary of the management of stroke and cerebral haemorrhage.

- Give oxygen via a mask.
- Assess the patient's level of consciousness using the Glasgow Coma Scale (*see* p. 43). Drowsiness is unusual in a stroke, and should raise the suspicion of cerebral haemorrhage. If this is the case, check the airway, place the patient in the recovery position, and call for help from senior colleagues.
- Keep the patient NBM until a swallow assessment has been done to assess the risk of aspiration. Commence IV fluids to prevent dehydration.
- An urgent CT scan of the head should be performed if haemorrhagic stroke is suspected. If cerebral haemorrhage is not suspected clinically, a CT scan should ideally be performed within 24 hours of presentation.

Table 10   Clinical features of stroke classified according to vascular territory

Artery occluded	Clinical features	Area of brain damaged
Middle cerebral artery	Contralateral hemiplegia (mainly leg) Dysphagia Dysarthria Dysphasia	Parietal (and frontal) cortex Broca's area (expressive) and Wernicke's area (receptive)
Posterior cerebral artery	Homonymous hemianopia	Visual cortex (occipital lobe)
Vertebral or basilar arteries	Motor, cranial or sensory nerve deficits Impaired consciousness	Brainstem
	Homonymous hemianopia	Visual cortex
Anterior cerebral arteries	Contralateral hemiplegia (mainly face/arm) Higher cognitive dysfunction	Frontal lobes
Deep penetrating arteries	Purely motor, purely sensory, sensory and motor Visual field defects	Internal capsule (lacunar infarct)

- Aspirin 300 mg should be given, as it improves survival in patients with cerebral infarction if given early. However, current guidelines state that it should only be used after CT scanning has failed to demonstrate evidence of haemorrhage.
- Catheterise the patient, as they are likely to be immobile.
- The following non-urgent investigations need to be performed to look for the underlying cause of stroke:
  - carotid Doppler scanning
  - echocardiography
  - fasting serum glucose and lipids.
- Rehabilitation in a specialist stroke unit has been shown to improve outcome and reduce complications post-stroke.
- Thrombolysis with alteplase is being used in a few centres in the UK. It has been shown to improve long-term disability due to stroke, especially if given within 3 hours of the onset of symptoms.

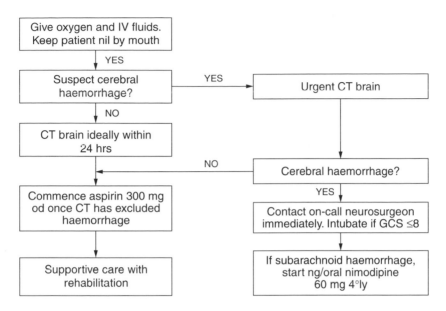

Figure 10 Integrated pathway for management of acute stroke and cerebral haemorrhage

Further reading

- Stroke Working Party of Royal College of Physicians of London (2004) *National Clinical Guidelines for Stroke* (2e). Royal College of Physicians of London, London.
- Schellinger PD, Kaste M and Hacke W (2004) An update on thrombolytic therapy for acute stroke. *Curr Opin Neurol.* **17**: 69–77.

Cerebral haemorrhage

Cerebral haemorrhage causes acute focal or global impairment of cerebral function, and may therefore mimic a stroke clinically. However, its management is very different, and the associated mortality is much higher than for stroke.

Subarachnoid haemorrhage

Subarachnoid haemorrhage (SAH) originates from the rupture of a berry aneurysm within the arterial circle of Willis. Blood enters the subarachnoid space, causing meningeal irritation, which in turn leads to photophobia, neck stiffness and a severe, occipital headache of sudden onset.

Intracerebral haemorrhage

Intracerebral haemorrhage is the most lethal type of stroke, with a mortality of 80%. It results from the rupture of Charcot–Bouchard microaneurysms which form in the brain parenchyma as a result of chronic hypertension. Intracerebral haemorrhage presents with sudden onset of features of raised intracranial pressure, such as impaired consciousness, nausea/vomiting, headache and papilloedema. Focal neurological deficits may also be seen, either via direct tissue damage or as false localising signs (*see* p. 46).

Subdural haemorrhage

Subdural haemorrhage is caused by the tearing of veins within the subdural space, and is almost always a consequence of head trauma. Since bleeding is venous rather than arterial, symptoms may take several days or even weeks to develop. The patient may initially present with agitation or confusion, and later exhibit features of raised intracranial pressure and focal neurological deficits.

Acute management of cerebral haemorrhage

Factors which should alert you to the presence of a cerebral haemorrhage include the following:

- drowsiness as assessed by the Glasgow Coma Scale (GCS) (*see* p. 43)
- features of meningism
- other features of raised intracranial pressure, such as papilloedema, false localising signs, nausea or vomiting.

If cerebral haemorrhage is suspected, take the following steps.

- *Give high-flow oxygen via a mask.*
- If the GCS score is ≤ 8, the patient cannot safely maintain their airway. In this case, the patient should be placed in the recovery position, and the on-call anaesthetist should be contacted at once for consideration of intubation.
- *Withhold aspirin, as this drug will increase the propensity for bleeding.*
- Keep the patient NBM and start IV fluids.
- Arrange an urgent CT scan of the head. Speak to senior colleagues if you have difficulty convincing the on-call radiologist!
- If subarachnoid haemorrhage is demonstrated, commence oral nimodipine 60 mg 4-hourly.
- *All patients with haemorrhagic stroke should be urgently referred to a neurosurgical team for treatment.*

For a summary of the management of cerebral haemorrhage, *see* Figure 10 (p. 53) in the previous section.

Further reading

- Stroke Working Party of the Royal College of Physicians of London (2004) *National Clinical Guidelines for Stroke* (2e). Royal College of Physicians of London, London.

Status epilepticus

A seizure (fit) is a sudden, transient alteration of neurological function, which may be either generalised (loss of consciousness) or partial (no loss of consciousness). Most seizures terminate spontaneously. However, the persistence of a seizure beyond 30 minutes, or recurrent seizures without recovery of consciousness between them, is defined as *status epilepticus*. Prompt treatment of these patients is vital in order to prevent hypoxic brain damage.

Clinical features

The most common type of generalised seizure is a tonic–clonic seizure, which may present with the following:

- a visual aura may precede the seizure
- limb jerking
- incontinence of urine and/or faeces
- tongue biting
- post-ictal state of coma or reduced consciousness for a few hours.

Causes of seizures

Seizures may occur as part of epilepsy, but in the hospital setting they are most likely to be due to a predisposing pathology such as the following:

- stroke or cerebral ischaemia (e.g. post-cardiac arrest)
- a space-occupying lesion such as a tumour, haemorrhage or brain abscess
- infection, such as meningitis or encephalitis (infection of the brain parenchyma)
- metabolic disturbances, such as:
    - hypoglycaemia (e.g. diabetes mellitus, alcoholism, malnutrition)
    - hypo/hypernatraemia
    - hypocalcaemia (e.g. hypoparathyroidism, osteomalacia)
    - hypomagnesaemia
    - liver failure, renal failure
- drugs, such as:
    - alcohol and other drugs of abuse
    - psychotropic drugs (e.g. phenothiazines, tricyclic antidepressants)
    - antibiotics (e.g. penicillin, isoniazid)
- vasculitis (e.g. systemic lupus erythematosus).

Initial management of any seizure

- The principles of basic life support (BLS) should be used. Check the airway, breathing and circulation (ABC). However, do not put your finger inside the patient's mouth during a seizure, as involuntary closure of the mouth may occur.
- Prevent injury to the patient by moving them away from any hazard such as furniture. It is important to hold and support the head in order to prevent it from hitting the ground during the seizure.
- Most seizures terminate spontaneously or with rectal diazepam which should be given immediately. However, if the seizure persists, further steps should be instituted (see below).
- After a seizure, the patient will be post-ictal, and will therefore be unconscious or drowsy. Re-check ABC, and then put the patient in the recovery position in order to prevent aspiration.

Further management of a seizure

Treatment is given in order to terminate, find the cause of and prevent damage due to the seizure. The management steps are as follows.

- high-flow oxygen via a face mask with a re-breathe bag to prevent hypoxia
- IV access and 10 mg IV or rectal diazepam
- give 250 mg IV thiamine if alcoholism is suspected, to prevent Wernicke's encephalopathy
- blood glucose monitoring (BM) stix for blood glucose measurement (give 50 ml 50% dextrose if the patient is hypoglycaemic, i.e. BM < 3.5 mM)
- urgent serum biochemistry for glucose, sodium, urea and electrolytes, liver function tests, calcium and magnesium, and immediate correction intravenously if any of the results are abnormal
- further diazepam 10 mg after 5 minutes if the seizure persists
- measurement of arterial blood gases to monitor for hypoxia
- intravenous phenytoin (loading dose of 15 mg/kg and maintenance dose of 100 mg 6- to 8-hourly, with monitoring of the plasma drug concentration) may terminate the seizure, but cardiac monitoring is essential during the administration of this drug because of the risk of tachyarrhythmias
- if the seizure persists after phenytoin administration or if, despite oxygen therapy, hypoxia is present, immediate anaesthetic assessment for intubation and transfer to intensive care are required

- after termination of the seizure, a brain CT or MRI scan (to look for evidence of stroke, tumour or haemorrhage) and lumbar puncture (if meningitis is suspected) may be needed.

Further reading

- British Medical Association and Royal Pharmaceutical Society of Great Britain (2004) Central nervous system. In: *British National Formulary 48*. British Medical Association and Royal Pharmaceutical Society of Great Britain, London.
- Delanty N, Vaughan CJ and French JA (1998) Medical causes of seizures. *The Lancet*. **352**: 1390.

4 Renal conditions

Acute renal failure

Acute renal failure (ARF) is the acute impairment of renal function, defined arbitrarily by a serum creatinine concentration greater than 200 micromol/l.

Causes of ARF

Broadly speaking, there are three categories of ARF.

- *Pre-renal failure* is by far the commonest cause of ARF in the hospital setting (> 90% of cases). It is caused by renal hypoperfusion in sepsis or hypotension/ shock.
- *Intrinsic renal disease* is the least common cause. It has various causes, including drugs (e.g.NSAIDs), infection and primary immunological disorders, and histologically it produces either glomerulonephritis or tubulo-interstitial nephritis.
- *Post-renal disorders* are caused by obstruction of renal outflow by calculi, prostatic hypertrophy or tumour.

Clinical features

Patients often present with non-specific symptoms such as nausea/ vomiting or tiredness. They may also complain of dyspnoea, orthopnoea and paroxysmal nocturnal dyspnoea, due to fluid overload. On examination, the following may be found:

- confusion
- a lemon-yellow tinge to the skin, and pruritus caused by uraemia
- fluid overload – raised JVP, peripheral oedema, bi-basal crackles (pulmonary oedema), ascites
- oliguria (although ARF may less commonly produce polyuria)
- pericardial rub.

Investigations

When the diagnosis of ARF has been established by measurement of urea and electrolytes, the following investigations should be performed:

- insertion of a urinary catheter and strict monitoring of fluid balance
- ECG to look for changes of hyperkalaemia (e.g. prolonging of the P-R interval, tall 'tented' T-waves and eventually a sinusoidal QRS complex and asytole)
- renal ultrasound examination to exclude urinary tract obstruction
- urinalysis:
  - microscopy (red cell casts indicate glomerulonephritis)
  - culture (to detect pyelonephritis)
  - Bence–Jones protein (to detect myeloma)
  - 24-hour collection for creatinine clearance
  - 24-hour collection for protein (> 3 g in nephrotic syndrome)
- serum immunology for anti-nuclear antibody (ANA), double-stranded DNA (dsDNA), anti-neutrophilic cytoplasmic antibodies (ANCA), complement and anti-glomerular membrane antibody
- serum biochemistry:
  - albumin (levels are low in nephrotic syndrome)
  - elevated creatine kinase (CK) and phosphate levels, and lowered calcium levels (indicate rhabdomyolysis)
  - protein electrophoresis (look for paraproteinaemia of myeloma).

Management

Pre-renal failure

The majority of cases of ARF are due to renal hypoperfusion. In such cases the patient will be hypotensive and/or show signs of dehydration, such as cool peripheries, capillary refill taking longer than 2 seconds, and dry mucous membranes. Give the patient normal saline (or colloid if they are hypotensive). After a few hours this should lead to recovery of renal function associated with initial polyuria. Take care to replace fluids adequately during this polyuric phase.

Pulmonary oedema

Patients may be fluid overloaded if they are olguric/anuric with a high fluid intake. Such patients may therefore develop pulmonary oedema causing respiratory distress.

- Give high-flow oxygen.
- Immediately stop any IV fluids, as these will worsen the fluid overload.
- Measure ABG.
- Commence IV GTN infusion (50 mg in 50 ml of normal saline at 0.5 to 10 mg/hour, increasing to a maximum dose with systolic blood pressure > 90 mmHg) to decrease pre-load to the heart.
- Give IV frusemide 40 mg to induce diuresis. Give a further 40 mg if there is no response.
- Continuous positive airways pressure (CPAP) is a mode of non-invasive ventilation which in the short term relieves pulmonary oedema.
- Negative fluid balance should be achieved in order to treat fluid overload.

Hyperkalaemia

A potassium concentration of > 6.8 mM or hyperkalaemia in the presence of typical ECG changes requires urgent treatment (see p. 62).

Indications for acute haemodialysis

Although most cases of ARF are treated conservatively, the renal team should be contacted in order to arrange acute haemodialysis if the patient has any of the following:

- severe hyperkalaemia (see above)
- pulmonary oedema that is refractory to conservative treatment
- encephalopathy
- pericarditis (high risk of tamponade).

Further reading

- Allbright RC Jr (2001) Acute renal failure: a practical update. *Mayo Clin Proc.* **76**: 67–74.

Hyperkalaemia

Hyperkalaemia (raised serum potassium levels) is a medical emergency as it may rapidly lead to asystolic cardiac arrest. Urgent treatment is indicated if the serum potassium concentration is higher than 6.8 mM or if ECG changes of hyperkalaemia are present.

Causes of hyperkalaemia

These include the following:

- acute renal failure (accounts for the majority of cases)
- rhabdomyolysis (raised CK and phosphate levels, and lowered calcium levels)
- tumour lysis syndrome (increased cell turnover during chemotherapy, particularly with haematological malignancies)
- drugs (e.g. ACE inhibitors).

Management

Hyperkalaemia requires urgent treatment if the potassium concentration is > 6.8 mM or in the presence of ECG changes. Otherwise, monitor potassium levels at least daily.

- Blood investigations:
  - U&Es (to detect acute renal failure)
  - bicarbonate concentration (low in acute renal failure)
  - CK, phosphate and calcium levels (to detect rhabdomyolysis)
  - urate levels (raised in tumour lysis syndrome).
- ECG – to detect changes of hyperkalaemia:
  - tall 'tented' T-waves
  - flat P-waves
  - broadening of the QRS complex (and eventually a sinusoidal QRS complex and asytole).
- Treatment of hyperkalaemia:
  - give 10 ml of 10% IV calcium gluconate to protect the myocardium from the effects of hyperkalaemia
  - also give 15 units of insulin with 50% dextrose over 30 minutes (with blood glucose monitoring), which *only temporarily* corrects hyperkalaemia by intracellular movement of K^+ ions
  - salbutamol nebulisers (5 mg) given regularly will temporarily lower serum potassium levels

- use calcium resonium (an ion-exchange resin administered orally or rectally), which lowers potassium levels, but only after several hours.
- Further management:
  - insert a urinary catheter and monitor fluid balance strictly
  - recheck U&Es and obtain a repeat ECG regularly
  - investigate and treat any coexisting acute renal failure (*see* p. 59)
  - call the renal team to arrange for urgent dialysis if the hyperkalaemia fails to improve.

Further reading

- Ahee P and Crowe AV (2000) The management of hyperkalaemia in the emergency department. *J Accid Emerg Med.* **17**: 188–91.

Rhabdomyolysis

Rhabdomyolysis is an acute metabolic disorder caused by widespread skeletal muscle damage and necrosis. Damaged myocytes release large amounts of myoglobin and potassium into the bloodstream, which may lead to acute renal failure and cardiac dysfunction if left untreated.

Causes of rhabdomyolysis

These include the following:

- trauma (e.g. resulting from a road traffic accident)
- excessive exercise (e.g. running the marathon when unfit)
- prolonged immobility
- prolonged seizure
- drugs (e.g. statins, malignant neuroleptic syndrome, ecstasy abuse).

Diagnosis of rhabdomyolysis

The patient may complain of tender muscles, the passage of dark, 'cola'-coloured urine or oliguria. They are usually febrile. The following classic blood results are found:

- substantially elevated CK levels – up to 1 million U/litre
- substantially elevated potassium levels
- elevated phosphate levels
- lowered calcium levels.

In addition, the serum urea and creatinine may become raised.

Management

Call senior colleagues as soon as you suspect rhabdomyolysis.

- Urinalysis will be positive for blood (since it cannot distinguish myoglobin from blood).
- Urine microscopy will demonstrate myoglobin.
- Measure ABG, which will demonstrate a metabolic acidosis.
- Stop all NSAIDs, as they will worsen any renal failure.
- Commence IV fluid resuscitation with normal saline.
- If the serum potassium concentration is > 6.8 mM or there are ECG changes of hyperkalaemia (e.g. tall 'tented' T-waves, flat P-waves,

broadening of QRS complex), give treatment for hyperkalaemia urgently (*see* p. 62).

- Catheterise the patient and closely monitor their urine output. Avoid the use of furosemide to achieve diuresis, as it promotes the precipitation of myoglobin in renal tubules.
- Alkaline diuresis may be indicated in order to stabilise the oxidised form of myoglobin and prevent it from causing damage to the renal tubules.
- The renal team should be asked to assess the need for acute dialysis if the patient becomes oliguric despite fluid resuscitation, or if they are hyperkalaemic despite treatment.
- Contact the on-call surgeons about the possible debridement of any necrotic tissue if the cause of rhabdomyolysis is trauma.

5 Endocrine conditions

Diabetic ketoacidosis

Diabetic ketoacidosis (DKA) occurs predominantly in type 1 diabetic patients as a result of inadequate insulin administration. The lack of insulin prevents the entry of glucose into cells, thus leading to the production of ketones and a metabolic acidosis. Furthermore, the extracellular hyperglycaemia leads to dehydration via osmotic diuresis.

Precipitating factors

These include the following:

- non-compliance with insulin
- infection
- pregnancy
- pancreatitis
- alcoholism.

Clinical features

Evidence of dehydration

- Hypotension.
- Low JVP.
- Dry mucous membranes.
- Capillary refill taking longer than 2 seconds.

Evidence of acidosis

- Tachypnoea.
- Kussmaul's breathing.

Evidence of precipitants of DKA

- Abdominal pain (think of pregnancy, pancreatitis, urinary tract infection and gastroenteritis).
- Cough, sputum (think of chest infection).
- Neck stiffness, headache, photophobia (think of meningitis).

Management

- Call for help from senior colleagues. It is important that they supervise the management of DKA.
- Obtain IV access.
- Measure ABG.
- Check the glucose stix reading.
- Give 10 IU Actrapid insulin subcutaneously immediately, and then commence an insulin sliding scale (50 IU Actrapid insulin in 50 ml normal saline) using the regime suggested in Table 11. (Note: the insulin infusion rate must *never* be zero, even if the glucose stix readings are normal, otherwise the DKA will only worsen. Therefore the minimum infusion rate on the sliding scale is 0.5 ml/hour.)

Table 11   Suggested insulin sliding scale for use in DKA

Glucose stix reading	Rate of Actrapid insulin administration (IU/hour)
0–4	0.5
4.1–7	2
7.1–11	3
11.1–14	4
14.1–17	5
> 17	6

- Aggressive IV fluid replacement is crucial, as these patients are so dehydrated. Follow the fluid regime suggested in Table 12.

Table 12   Suggested fluid regimen for DKA (note that the serum potassium concentration must be measured every few hours using ABG)

Bag of fluid to be infused	Duration of infusion (hours)	Type of fluid
First litre	0.5	Normal saline + 20 mmol KCl
Second litre	1	Normal saline + 20 mmol KCl
Third litre	1.5	Normal saline + 20 mmol KCl
Fourth litre	2	Normal saline + 20 mmol KCl
Fifth litre	4	Normal saline + 20 mmol KCl

- ABG should be measured every few hours in order to monitor the serum potassium level (which may fall rapidly when insulin is given) and the improvement in acidosis.
- Once the glucose concentration is below 12 mM, the maintenance fluid should be switched to 5% dextrose, so that more insulin can be administered, thereby accelerating the reversal of ketoacidosis.
- The patient should be catheterised, and urine output should be monitored closely.
- The following investigations should be performed:
  - send blood for a full blood count, clotting factors, U&Es, LFTs, amylase and blood cultures
  - measure the urinary human chorionic gonadotropin (HCG) concentration to rule out pregnancy
  - dipstick and send urine for culture
  - send sputum for culture
  - take a chest X-ray
  - perform an ECG.
- If the patient is hypotensive, oliguric or acidotic with no response to treatment, central venous access should be obtained and intensive care should be considered.
- Sliding-scale insulin should be continued until the patient is eating and drinking and the urine is free of ketones (as measured by multistix).

The management of diabetic ketoacidosis is summarised in Figure 11.

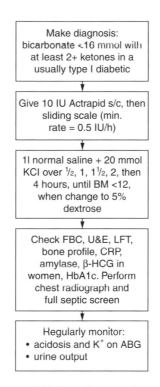

Make diagnosis:
bicarbonate <16 mmol with
at least 2+ ketones in a
usually type I diabetic

↓

Give 10 IU Actrapid s/c, then
sliding scale (min.
rate = 0.5 IU/h)

↓

1l normal saline + 20 mmol
KCl over ½, 1, 1½, 2, then
4 hours, until BM <12,
when change to 5%
dextrose

↓

Check FBC, U&E, LFT,
bone profile, CRP,
amylase, β-HCG in
women, HbA1c. Perform
chest radiograph and
full septic screen

↓

Regularly monitor:
• acidosis and K⁺ on ABG
• urine output

Figure 11   Management of diabetic ketoacidosis

Further reading

● Bassett D, Dornhorst A, McHardy-Young S *et al.* (eds) (2002) Diabetic ketoacidosis. In: *Hammersmith Hospitals NHS Trust Guidelines for the Management of Diabetes Mellitus*; www.meeran.info

Hyper-osmolar non-ketotic acidosis

Hyper-osmolar non-ketotic acidosis (HONK) is caused by persistently raised serum glucose levels in a patient with type 2 diabetes. The osmotic diuresis of glycosuria leads to severe, life-threatening dehydration. However, the presence of insulin in these patients prevents ketoacidosis.

Diagnostic features

The following features help to distinguish HONK from diabetic ketoacidosis:

- osmolality > 320 Osmol/litre (serum osmolality = ($[Na^+]$ + $[K^+]$) × 2 + [glucose] + [urea])
- urinary ketones negative or 1+
- blood glucose concentration in the range 40–100 mmol/litre
- bicarbonate concentration > 16 mmol/litre.

Precipitating factors

- Non-compliance with insulin.
- Infection.
- Pregnancy.
- Pancreatitis.
- Alcoholism.

Clinical features

Look for evidence of severe dehydration, including the following:

- hypotension
- low JVP
- dry mucous membranes
- capillary refill taking more than 2 seconds
- oliguria or anuria.

In addition, there may be signs of infection, and the patient may be confused or drowsy.

Management

- Obtain IV access.
- Monitor ABG.
- Check the glucose stix reading.
- Give 10 IU of Actrapid insulin subcutaneously immediately.

The following investigations should be performed.

- Send blood for FBC, clotting, LFTs, osmolality, amylase, blood cultures and U&Es (be alert for pseudohyponatraemia, in which the sodium concentration appears falsely low due to the presence of high serum glucose levels).
- Measure the urinary HCG concentration in order to rule out pregnancy.
- Dipstick and send urine for culture.
- Send sputum for culture.
- Take a chest X-ray.
- If necessary, perform a CT scan and then a lumbar puncture (if there is no focal intracranial lesion).

Further management

- Rapid correction of serum osmolality leads to cerebral oedema. Therefore the central aim of treatment is to *slowly* correct the osmolality (i.e. by no more than 5 mOsmol/litre/kg/hour). The key to achieving this is the fluid and insulin regime given to the patient.
  - Start an insulin sliding scale (50 IU Actrapid insulin in 50 ml normal saline) using a regime such as that shown in Table 13. Note that lower than normal doses of insulin are used in order to prevent rapid changes in serum glucose concentration, and therefore serum osmolality.
  - Initially use normal saline as fluid replacement, as this has a higher osmolality than 5% dextrose, so it will reduce serum osmolality more slowly. Give the first litre over 2 hours, a further litre over 4 hours, and then another over 8 hours. Add potassium to fluids from the second bag, but check the serum potassium concentration at least three times in the first 24 hours to ensure that there is correct replacement. Only when the blood glucose concentration is < 12 mM should fluid replacement be switched to 5% dextrose.
- The patient should be catheterised, and urine output should be monitored closely.

Table 13   Suggested insulin sliding scale for use in HONK

Glucose stix reading	Rate of Actrapid insulin administration (IU/hour)
0–4	0
4.1–7	1
7.1–12	2
> 12	3

- Make sure that the patient is anti-coagulated with subcutaneous enoxaparin 40 mg daily if there is normal renal function, or with subcutaneous heparin 5000 IU twice daily if there is renal failure.
- If the patient is hypotensive or oliguric, central venous access should be obtained and intensive care should be considered.

The management of hyper-osmolar non-ketotic acidosis is summarised in Figure 12.

Further reading

- Bassett D, Dornhorst A, McHardy-Young S *et al.* (eds) (2002) Hyper-osmolar non-ketotic acidosis. In: *Hammersmith Hospitals NHS Trust Guidelines for the Management of Diabetes Mellitus*; www.meeran.info

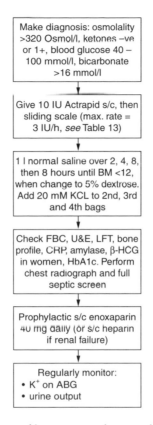

Figure 12   Management of hyper-osmolar non-ketotic acidosis

Hypoglycaemia

Hypoglycaemia is defined as a serum glucose concentration of less than 3.6 mM, and severe hypoglycaemia as a serum glucose concentration of less than 2.2 mM. Coma, seizures and death may all occur if hypoglycaemia is left untreated.

Causes of hypoglycaemia

The commonest cause of hypoglycaemia is accidental over-administration of insulin or sulphonylureas such as gliclazide or glibeclamide for diabetes mellitus. Other causes include the following:

- alcoholism
- chronic liver disease
- renal failure – the insulin requirement for diabetic patients decreases in renal failure due to its renal clearance
- abuse of insulin or sulphonylureas, especially by healthcare professionals such as nurses
- other drugs (e.g. salicylates, quinine)
- adrenal insufficiency (*see* p. 78) or hypopituitarism
- insulinoma (extremely rare).

Clinical features

Hypoglycaemia is a potent stimulant of the sympathetic nervous system. Therefore patients typically develop the following:

- hunger
- irritability
- tachycardia
- tremor
- sweating
- pallor.

More severe hypoglycaemia may also produce neuroglycopenia, with the following features:

- blurred vision
- drowsiness or coma
- seizure.

Diabetic patients who frequently have hypoglycaemic attacks may develop hypoglycaemic unawareness, which is loss of the features of hypoglycaemia caused by sympathetic stimulation. This is extremely dangerous, as neuroglycopenia develops without warning.

Management

- If hypoglycaemia is suspected, blood glucose levels should initially be monitored with BM stix and a glucometer.
- If the patient is unresponsive, put them in the recovery position to protect their airway.
- Obtain IV access with a large-bore cannula.
- Send venous blood samples for measurement of glucose (to confirm hypoglycaemia), urea and electrolytes and liver function tests (to screen for secondary causes of hypoglycaemia).
- Send blood samples for measurement of insulin and C-peptide if you suspect abuse of insulin. (Endogenous insulin leads to a rise in both insulin and C-peptide, but injected insulin only leads to a rise in insulin.) Send blood and urine samples for a sulphonylurea screen if you suspect the abuse of this drug.
- If alcoholism is suspected, 250 mg IV thiamine must be given *prior* to glucose (as glucose may precipitate Wernicke's encephalopathy).
- If the patient is able to take oral fluids, give them a sweet drink such as Lucozade.
- If the patient is drowsy, give them 25–50 ml of 50% dextrose, and monitor for rapid clinical improvement.
- If IV access cannot be obtained, give 1 mg IM glucagon. However, glucose must be given orally as soon as possible (before the effects of the glucagon wear off).

Further reading

- Bassett D, Dornhorst A, McHardy-Young S *et al.* (eds) (2002) *Hammersmith Hospitals NHS Trust Guidelines for the Management of Diabetes Mellitus*; www.meeran.info

Phaeochromocytoma

Phaeochromocytoma is a tumour of the adrenal medulla (or any sympathetic ganglion) which is characterised by excessive secretion of catecholamines such as adrenaline (epinephrine), noradrenaline (norepinephrine) and dopamine. Around 10% of phaeochromocytoma cases are bilateral, 10% are extra-adrenal and 10% are malignant. Phaeochromocytoma causes hypertension mediated by α_1-adrenergic vasoconstriction. Tachycardia also occurs and is mediated via the positively inotropic effect of stimulation of β_1-adrenergic receptors in the heart.

Clinical features

The patient may give a history of *paroxysmal* symptoms such as palpitations, anxiety/panic attacks or poorly controlled hypertension. Look for the following signs:

- hypertension
- sweating
- peripheral vasoconstriction
- tachycardia
- arrhythmias
- evidence of acute cardiac failure.

Precipitants of phaeochromocytoma crisis

- Unopposed β-blockade (use of a β-blocker).
- General anaesthetic.
- IV radiological contrast.
- Drugs (e.g. opiates, tricyclic antidepressants, metoclopramide).

Principles of management

- Always seek help from senior colleagues immediately if phaeochromocytoma is suspected.
- Do not wait for confirmation of the diagnosis of phaeochromocytoma before initiating treatment, as any delay in treatment could prove fatal! Treatment may be later discontinued if subsequent investigations exclude the diagnosis.

- Since affected individuals are heavily fluid depleted due to long-standing vasoconstriction, α-blockade may precipitate potentially fatal hypotension unless the dehydration is corrected first.
- Never give the patient a β-blocker until they are fully α-blocked. This is because the hypertension associated with phaeochromocytoma will worsen on removal of the vasodilatory action of β_2-receptors which oppose the action of α-receptors.

Management pathway

- A central line is usually needed to monitor fluid status.
- Give large volumes of intravenous fluids prior to α-blockade to prevent hypotension.
- Administer a bolus (0.5–5 mg) of IV phentolamine followed by an infusion of IV phentolamine. This is a short-acting, competitive α-blocker that antagonises the vasoconstriction caused by catecholamines released from the tumour.
- In order to achieve full (non-competitive/irreversible) α-blockade, IV phenoxybenzamine 0.5 mg/kg should be given daily for 3 days.
- *Do not stop IV phentolamine infusion until IV phenoxybenzamine has been given for 3 days*, when full α-blockade is achieved. Thereafter, the patient should be continued on oral phenoxybenzamine.
- β-blockade (e.g. with atenolol) may be given to treat tachycardia only after 3 days of intravenous phenoxybenzamine. β-blockers must never be given until the patient is fully α-blocked (see above).
- The diagnosis of phaeochromocytoma should only be made when the patient has completely recovered from the acute illness (to avoid false-positive test results).
  - Send three 24-hour urine collections for measurement of catecholamines, the levels of which are raised in phaeochromocytoma.
  - If urine catecholamines are equivocal, contact the endocrine team to discuss performing a pentolinium or clonidine suppression test.
  - CT and MRI scans and meta-iodobiguanide (MIBG) nuclear scintigraphy may be used to localise the tumour.

Addisonian crisis

Addison's disease is a condition caused by a deficiency in the production of glucocorticoids (mainly cortisol) and possibly mineralocorticoids (mainly aldosterone) from the adrenal cortex. The term 'Addisonian crisis' describes the clinical state that may arise as a result of adrenal insufficiency. Since long-term steroid treatment leads to adrenal suppression, individuals who are receiving such treatment are also susceptible to Addisonian crisis.

Aetiology of Addison's disease

Most cases of Addison's disease are due to autoimmune destruction of the adrenal cortex (primary Addison's). Other causes of adrenal destruction include the following:

- tuberculosis
- metastatic carcinoma, lymphoma
- haemorrhage associated with meningococcal septicaemia (Waterhouse–Friedrichsen syndrome).

Secondary adrenal failure arises from impairment of adrenocorticotropic hormone (ACTH) secretion (e.g. due to a pituitary tumour or cranial irradiation).

Precipitants of Addisonian crisis

The following factors may trigger Addisonian crisis in individuals with adrenal insufficiency or adrenal suppression:

- inadequate steroid replacement dose
- sudden cessation of long-term steroid treatment (e.g. for severe asthma)
- infection
- major surgery
- any serious illness.

Clinical features

The patient may give a recent history consistent with Addison's disease, including symptoms such as tiredness, dizziness, nausea and vomiting. Alternatively, there may be a history of chronic oral steroid treatment (e.g. for severe asthma). On examination the patient may show any of the following features:

- hypotension
- postural hypotension (a fall in systolic blood pressure > 15 mmHg on moving from lying to standing position)
- drowsiness or decreased consciousness
- increased pigmentation (in primary adrenal failure, due to increased ACTH secretion)
- seizure
- they may be wearing a 'steroid bracelet' stating that they are on long-term steroids.

Management

- It is vital to give steroids (IV hydrocortisone 200 mg) *immediately* if you suspect Addisonian crisis! If in doubt, give hydrocortisone anyway, since the risk of not treating Addisonian crisis far outweighs any risk of giving an unnecessary dose of steroids.
- Remember to look for clues that someone is likely to be steroid dependent:
  - history of long-term steroid usage
  - history of a chronic, steroid-treatable condition such as inflammatory bowel disease or asthma
  - steroid bracelet
  - cushingoid appearance.
- Serum sodium and bicarbonate levels tend to be low. Serum potassium levels are classically high.
- Measure the blood glucose concentration, looking for evidence of hypoglycaemia.
- Establish IV access.
- Administer fluid resuscitation. If the patient is hypotensive, give IV colloid (e.g. gelofusine) rapidly until they are normotensive. However, if the patient is normotensive, normal saline may be given.
- The Synacthen test is used to diagnose Addison's disease. Plasma cortisol is measured before and 30 and 60 minutes after injection of Synacthen, a synthetic ACTH analogue. In Addison's disease, plasma cortisol levels at 60 minutes are low (< 550 nM) and/or there is an inadequate rise (< 180 nM) from the baseline measurement.
- Send sputum, urine and blood samples and wound swabs for culture. Consider giving empirical antibiotics if there is evidence of sepsis (e.g. pyrexia).

- Long-term steroid replacement for Addison's disease consists of oral hydrocortisone given two to three times per day together with once-daily fludrocortisone.

Further reading

- Turner H and Wass J (2002) Adrenal disorders. In: *Oxford Handbook of Endocrinology and Diabetes*. Oxford University Press, Oxford.

6 Haematology/ oncology

Deep vein thrombosis

Thromboembolic disease is the third commonest cause of death in hospitalised patients in the UK. It usually arises as thrombosis in a deep leg vein, known as deep vein thrombosis (DVT). This detaches and comes to rest in the pulmonary artery, when it is termed a pulmonary embolism (PE) (*see* p. 83).

Predisposing factors

- Immobility.
- Major surgery (particularly orthopaedic).
- Smoking.
- Pregnancy or the oral contraceptive pill.
- Malignancy.
- Haematological conditions (especially myeloma).
- Vasculitis (e.g. systemic lupus erythematosus).
- Thrombophilia (e.g. protein C deficiency, anti-phospholipid syndrome).

Clinical features

DVT can be 'silent' (i.e. asymptomatic) or it can present with calf pain, typically in the second post-operative week. On examination the calf is hot, swollen and tender, and the pain is worsened by ankle plantar flexion (Homan's sign). The patient is often also systemically unwell and pyrexial. If the pelvic or femoral veins are affected, the poor venous drainage causes swelling of the entire lower limb.

Doppler ultrasound scanning is a simple, non-invasive, reliable method of diagnosing DVT in veins above the knee. For the calf and smaller DVT it is difficult to visualise thrombi by Doppler scanning, even with duplex techniques. However, the significance of below-knee DVT, which is thought to be present in over 70% of post-operative patients, is controversial, and as a result the condition is most often not treated.

Management

Anticoagulant therapy with subcutaneous low-molecular-weight heparin or IV fractionated heparin will both help to prevent further clot propagation and increase fibrinolysis. Once the patient has been fully anticoagulated, heparin therapy is replaced by oral warfarin treatment. It is important to remember that during the immediate post-operative period, anticoagulant therapy may increase the risk of significant haemorrhage, and should therefore not be instituted without advice from senior colleagues. If bleeding does occur in treated patients, protamine sulphate can be used to reverse the effect of unfractionated heparin, but has no effect on low-molecular-weight heparin.

Further reading

- Lopez JA, Kearon C and Lee AY (2004) Deep venous thrombosis. *Hematology.* 439–56.
- McRae SJ and Ginsberg JS (2004) Initial treatment of venous thromboembolism. *Circulation.* **110 (Suppl. 1):** I3–9.

Pulmonary embolism

Pulmonary embolism/embolus (PE) is one of the commonest complications of hospital admission in the UK. It is particularly common in the elderly, and has a high mortality.

The classic presentation of PE is an old man who feels suddenly short of breath after straining on the toilet. PE is also common in post-operative patients around day 10. The size of the pulmonary arterial vessel that is blocked by the PE will determine the severity of the condition, which can thus vary from mild symptoms of dyspnoea and mild pleuritic chest pain to sudden death from an occluded main pulmonary artery. Haemoptysis is a frequent symptom, as is confusion due to hypoxia in elderly patients.

Clinical features

On examination the patient may show any of the following:

- signs of DVT (e.g. swollen, red, painful leg) (*see* p. 81)
- tachycardia
- pleural rub.

If the PE is 'massive', the following signs of cardiovascular compromise with right-sided heart failure may be present:

- cyanosis
- hypotension (obstructive shock)
- raised jugulovenous pressure (JVP) with prominent 'A' wave
- left parasternal (right-ventricular) heave
- right-ventricular third heart sound (S3).

However, PE can occur in the absence of any obvious DVT and, as both myocardial infarction and chest infection can mimic its presentation, a very high index of suspicion is needed to make the diagnosis of PE. *Any post-operative or elderly immobile patient who appears unwell or confused, or who is recovering more slowly than would be expected, should have this diagnosis considered.*

Management

Patients with suspected PE should be treated empirically for this condition until the diagnosis has been either confirmed or excluded. Management therefore consists of the following:

- high-flow oxygen via a mask
- IV access with a large-bore cannula
- if the patient is hypotensive, give IV colloid
- ABG monitoring – lowered pO_2 sometimes with lowered pCO_2 and a respiratory alkalosis
- ECG may show:
  - sinus tachycardia (the commonest finding in PE)
  - T-wave inversion and/or ST changes anteriorly
  - new right bundle branch block
  - right axis deviation
  - S1 Q3 T3 (dominant S in lead I, Q waves in lead III, T-wave inversion in lead III) – although this is said to be a 'classical' finding, it only occurs in 15% of cases of PE
- chest X-ray – commonly clear, but may show a pleural effusion or a wedge-shaped area of consolidation (indicating pulmonary infarction)
- a non-steroidal anti-inflammatory drug (NSAID) such as ibuprofen to relieve any pleuritic pain
- anti-coagulation with low-molecular-weight heparin (e.g. enoxaparin 1.5 mg/kg every 24 hours).

Establishing the diagnosis of PE

- If the chest X-ray is clear, request a ventilation/perfusion (V/Q) scan.
- Otherwise request a spiral CT (CT pulmonary angiogram).
- A negative d-dimer (< 500 mcg/litre) suggests that PE is unlikely. However, it has a low specificity and it is uninterpretable in patients over the age of 80 years or after surgery. For these reasons it is now rarely performed.

Massive PE

PE with signs of right-sided heart failure or even cardiogenic shock has a very high associated mortality. Therefore two new techniques are increasingly being used to treat it.

- *Thrombolysis:* Recent trials have shown that thrombolysis may be more beneficial than anti-coagulation in patients with evidence of right-sided heart failure. However, the risk of cerebral haemorrhage may be up to 3%. Thrombolysis delivered via a pulmonary artery catheter may be associated with a lower risk of intracranial haemorrhage.
- *Pulmonary embolectomy:* Although practised by only a few cardiothoracic centres in the UK, embolectomy is a useful alternative to thrombolysis, particularly in patients at high risk of an intracranial haemorrhage.

Recurrent PE

Recurrent small PEs can lead to chronic pulmonary hypertension and should therefore be prevented by inserting an inferior vena caval filter (e.g. Greenfield filter) to 'catch' any propagating emboli that originate in the pelvic or femoral veins.

Further reading

- Goldhaber SZ (2002) Modern treatment of pulmonary embolism. *Eur Respir J Suppl.* **35**: 22–7s.
- Konstantinides S (2004) Should thrombolytic therapy be used in patients with pulmonary embolism? *Am J Cardiovasc Drugs.* **4**: 69–74.

Disseminated intravascular coagulopathy

Disseminated intravascular coagulopathy (DIC) is a haematological emergency which may result from one of a host of physiological insults. It is characterised by the aberrant activation of thrombotic pathways, which leads to excessive generation of thrombin. Clot deposition occurs in small blood vessels, and subsequently damages erythrocytes passing through these vessels (this condition is known as microangiopathic haemolytic anaemia, MAHA). Thus haemolysis, consumption of platelets and consumption of clotting factors occur simultaneously.

Aetiology

Almost any severe form of illness may cause DIC. However, the main causes are as follows:

- sepsis, especially involving Gram-negative organisms (e.g. meningococcus)
- acute pancreatitis
- blood group incompatibility following transfusion
- adenocarcinoma (e.g. lung, prostate)
- amniotic fluid embolus
- fat embolus.

Clinical features

Features of the underlying disease process may be evident. However, DIC itself may cause the following:

- bleeding (e.g. purpura, gastrointestinal bleeding, haemoptysis)
- cerebral microangiopathy (e.g. confusion, coma or seizures)
- acute renal failure via renal microangiopathy
- acute respiratory distress syndrome (ARDS).

Diagnosis

The diagnosis of DIC is suggested by the following test results:

- lowered Hb
- lowered platelet count
- lowered fibrinogen
- raised prothrombin time (PT)
- raised APTT (activated partial thromboplastin time)

- blood film demonstrates fragmented erythrocytes consistent with MAHA.

Management

Once the diagnosis of DIC has been made, management is directed at determination of the underlying cause, and prevention of complications such as bleeding and renal failure.

- Perform a full septic screen including blood, sputum, urine and wound cultures. Then start broad-spectrum antibiotics if sepsis is suspected.
- Measure the serum amylase to screen for acute pancreatitis, particularly if the patient has abdominal pain.
- Stop transfusion of any blood products and check that they are correct for your patient.
- Catheterise the patient, closely monitor urine output and check U&Es. If there is oliguria or acute renal impairment, central line insertion and central venous pressure (CVP) monitoring should be considered.
- Check LFTs and bicarbonate to look for evidence of liver dysfunction and acidosis, respectively.
- If there is any evidence of bleeding, liaise with the on-call haematologist to arrange urgent transfusion of platelets and cryoprecipitate (which is rich in factor VIII and fibrinogen).
- Further management of DIC should be guided by the advice of the on-call haematologist. Recent trials have demonstrated that recombinant activated protein kinase C may improve the outcome in sepsis-related DIC.

Further reading

- Toh CH and Dennis M (2003) Disseminated intravascular coagulation: old disease, new hope. *BMJ*. **327**: 974–7.

Neutropenic sepsis

Neutropenic sepsis is defined as a fever of $> 38°C$ in a patient with a neutrophil count of $< 1.0 \times 10^9$ cells/litre. Such patients are immunocompromised by the low neutrophil number and are therefore at increased risk of infection.

Aetiology of neutropenia

Common causes include the following:

- chemotherapy
- haematological conditions that cause bone-marrow destruction, such as:
    - leukaemia (lymphoproliferative or myeloproliferative)
    - myelodysplasia
    - multiple myeloma
- drugs (e.g. carbimazole)
- viral infection (e.g. human parvovirus)
- aplastic anaemia.

Aetiology of neutropenic sepsis

Bacterial infection accounts for most cases of neutropenic sepsis. Common causative organisms include the following:

- Gram-positive cocci (e.g. coagulase-negative staphylococci, *Staphylococcus aureus*, *Streptococcus viridans*)
- Gram-negative bacilli (e.g. *Escherichia coli*, *Klebsiella*, *Pseudomonas aeruginosa*).

Fungal infections such as aspergillosis and viral infections (e.g. cytomegalovirus (CMV), influenza) may also cause neutropenic sepsis.

Clinical features

It is of paramount importance to look *thoroughly* for the source of sepsis in a neutropenic patient. The following sites must be considered:

- chest (cough, shortness of breath, sputum)
- mouth (teeth, gums, pharynx)
- ear (otitis externa or media)

- gastrointestinal (vomiting, abdominal pain, diarrhoea) (Note: avoid performing a digital rectal examination before consulting senior colleagues about this, due to the risk of bacteraemia)
- cannulae or central lines (these should be changed immediately, and the line tips cultured)
- skin (cellulitis, and fungal, herpes and varicella zoster infections)
- urine
- ano-genital region (infection or discharge may indicate reactivation of genital herpes)
- CNS (evidence of meningitis or raised intracranial pressure)
- eyes (conjunctivitis, choriorctinitis, CMV, choroidoretinitis).

Management

- *Consult your hospital guidelines on the management of neutropenic sepsis.*
- Look thoroughly for the site of infection, which is often evident (*see* above).
- Start IV fluids and treat septic shock if present (*see* p 253)
- Send off blood for FBC and analysis of coagulation factors. Note: it is important to be alert for DIC, which is indicated by thrombocytopenia, progressive anaemia and impaired clotting with low fibrinogen levels.
- Send off samples for biochemical blood investigations such as U&Es, LFTs and CRP.
- Samples from potential sources of infection should be sent for microscopy and culture. These include the following:
  - sputum
  - stool, including *Clostridium difficile* toxin assay and microscopy for *Cryptosporidium* if the patient has diarrhoea
  - urinalysis and culture
  - blood cultures (peripheral and also through IV catheter lumens)
  - samples for mycobacterial blood culture should be sent in special culture bottles supplied by the laboratory if required
  - a CT scan followed by lumbar puncture should be performed if meningitis or encephalitis is suspected.
- A chest radiograph should be performed in all patients to look for evidence of pneumonia.
- Check your hospital protocol with regard to the choice of empirical antibiotic to be used. Table 14 shows one such protocol. If a likely source of infection is found, consult with the on-call microbiologist

and haematologist/oncologist for advice on any possible change in the choice of antibiotic.

- Always seek advice from the on-call haematologist/oncologist on further investigation into the cause of neutropenia and sepsis (if not already known), and the further management of your patient.
- Rapid deterioration can occur in neutropenic sepsis, so have a low threshold for calling the ITU for assessment if needed.

Table 14   Risk stratification of neutropenic patients and suggested choice of empirical antibiotics

Risk category of patient	Clinical features	Antibiotic regimen
High risk	Neutrophils < 0.5 × 10^9/litre	Imepenam (500 mg four times daily IV) or
	Comorbidity Immunosuppression with HIV or drugs (e.g. cyclosporin)	Tazosin (4.5 g three times daily IV) + gentamicin (3–5 mg/kg daily IV) if septic shock or pseudomonal infection likely
Low risk	Neutrophils 0.5–1.0 × 10^9/litre No septic shock	Oral or IV ciprofloxacin or augmentin

Further reading

- Taylor M, Anderson H, Mutton K *et al.* (2005) *Guidelines for the Management of Neutropenic Sepsis.* Christie Hospital, Manchester; www.christie.nhs.uk/neutropenic

Sickle-cell crisis

Sickle-cell anaemia results from a single point mutation in the haemo-globin β-chain. In homozygotes, the mutated haemoglobin (HbS) chain polymerises at low oxygen tensions, which leads to sickling of erythrocytes. This results in the occlusion of small blood vessels, which may in turn cause acute crises.

Trigger factors
- Hypoxia.
- Acidosis.
- Sepsis.
- Dehydration.

Vaso-occlusive crisis

The occlusion of small vessels supplying the bone marrow leads to severe bony pain. In children the hands and feet are predominantly involved, whereas in adults the vertebrae, femur, humerus and ribs are mainly involved. Clinical features include the following:

- severe bony pain
- tachycardia
- pyrexia.

Note that minor vaso-occlusive crises are common, and are often relieved by analgesia alone, without the need for hospital admission. However, severe cases may require management in hospital.

Sickle chest crisis

Infarction of the bone marrow from vaso-occlusive crises leads to the release of fat emboli, which may cause pulmonary infarction. Clinical features include the following:

- dyspnoea
- tachycardia
- pleural rub
- pleural effusion
- right-sided heart failure (hypotension, raised JVP, right ventricular heave, fourth heart sound).

Sequestration crisis

Occlusion of venous drainage from organs such as the spleen or liver leads to painful enlargement and subsequent chronic infarction. Most homozygous adults are therefore asplenic due to auto-infarction. Clinical features are as follows:

- painful and/or enlarged spleen
- painful and/or enlarged liver.

Aplastic crisis

Infection with human parvovirus B19 may cause marrow aplasia, leading to severe anaemia. Clinical features may include the following:

- tachycardia
- congestive cardiac failure (third heart sound, raised JVP, pulmonary oedema, peripheral oedema).

Management

- Give high-flow oxygen.
- Rehydrate the patient with IV normal saline (give the first litre over 2 hours).
- Treat painful crises with adequate analgesia. Often this will consist of substantial doses of opioids.
- Send blood samples for FBC, reticulocytes, group and save, U&Es and blood cultures.
- Monitor ABG, and obtain a chest X-ray and an ECG to look for evidence of sickle chest crisis.
- Give IV penicillin (or erythromycin if the patient is allergic to penicillin) to cover for capsulate infection (e.g. pneumococcus), which more commonly affects asplenic patients.
- If the patient complains of abdominal pain, obtain an abdominal radiograph, check the serum amylase and seek a surgical opinion if necessary.
- Transfusion of blood (which ideally should be fully genotyped) may be necessary to compensate for the severe anaemia associated with aplastic crisis.
- Seek advice from the on-call haematologist if the patient shows signs of shock, an acute abdomen or pulmonary embolism. Exchange transfusion (replacement of native blood with normal HbA blood) may be needed in life-threatening crises.

Further reading

- British Association for Accident and Emergency (1997) *Guidelines for the Management of Sickle-Cell Crises.* British Association for Accident and Emergency, London; www.baem.org.uk/sickle.htm

Acute transfusion reaction

In recent years the potential hazards associated with blood product administration have become an extremely important issue in medical practice. One of the most important ways of avoiding problems is to only prescribe blood products that are absolutely needed. In addition, strict protocols with regard to blood product labelling, collection and administration must be adhered to.

Classification of acute transfusion reactions

Fortunately, life-threatening acute transfusion reactions are rare. The vast majority of reactions are mild and resolve with conservative treatment (*see* Table 15).

Table 15 Classification of acute transfusion reactions

Non-severe acute transfusion reactions	*Severe acute transfusion reactions*
Acute febrile reaction Acute urticarial reaction	Acute haemolytic transfusion reaction/ABO incompatibility Infusion of a bacterially contaminated unit Transfusion-associated lung injury (TRALI) Severe allergic reaction or anaphylaxis

Clinical features

The following clinical features should alert you to the presence of an acute transfusion reaction:

- generally feeling unwell
- fever/rigors
- flushing
- nausea/vomiting
- urticaria
- bone, muscle, chest and/or abdominal pain
- hypertension or hypotension
- respiratory distress.

Management

- *Stop the transfusion of blood product immediately.* This is the single most important treatment you can give your patient.
- Re-check that the correct unit of blood is being given to the patient.
- If the only feature of a transfusion reaction is pyrexia < 38.5°C or an urticarial rash, the reaction is likely to be mild. It should be adequate to give paracetamol for fever, IV chlorpheniramine (chlorphenamine, 10 mg) for urticaria, and then recommence the transfusion at a slower rate. The patient should be closely monitored afterwards.
- If the patient's clinical features are more severe than pyrexia or urticaria, a severe transfusion reaction must be suspected. Repeat blood samples including group and save, FBC, blood film, clotting and U&Es should always be sent. In addition, it is important to liaise closely with the on-call haematologist and seek their advice.

Severe allergic reaction

Angioedema, wheeze, stridor and hypotension suggest a severe anaphylactic reaction.

- Return the transfused (and other cross-matched) blood products to the blood bank.
- Treat the patient for anaphylaxis with oxygen, salbutamol nebulisers, IV chlorpheniramine and IM (*not* IV) adrenaline (*see* p. 258).

ABO incompatibility

If it is discovered that the wrong unit of blood has been transfused to your patient, swift action is vital as DIC is likely to occur.

- Inform the blood bank of the incident and return the unit to the blood bank.
- Start an infusion of IV normal saline.
- Catheterise the patient and measure their hourly urine output. If oliguria occurs, consider central venous access.
- Re-send full bloods including FBC, blood film, clotting profile and U&Es. Beware of DIC as indicated by impaired clotting with falling platelet counts, haemoglobin and fibrinogen (*see* p. 86).
- Seek advice from senior colleagues on the requirement for ITU admission.

Infusion of a bacterially contaminated unit

If repeat bloods demonstrate haemolysis in the absence of blood incompatibility, the possibility of bacterial contamination should be considered. Management is as described above for ABO incompatibility (since these patients are at risk of DIC). However, broad-spectrum antibiotics should also be given.

Transfusion-associated lung injury (TRALI)

If severe dyspnoea occurs in the absence of features of anaphylaxis (i.e. wheeze or stridor), TRALI should be suspected. The patient normally has widespread coarse crackles. TRALI, which is a form of acute respiratory distress syndrome (ARDS), results in increased permeability of the alveolar membrane and thus pulmonary oedema.

- Give high-flow oxygen.
- Chest radiograph shows widespread interstitial shadowing.
- Check progress with ABG monitoring.
- Invasive ventilation in an ITU may be required.

Further reading

- Joint UK Blood Transfusion Services (2005) Management of acute transfusion reactions. In: *UK Blood Transfusion and Tissue Transplantation Guidelines*; www.transfusionguidelines.org.uk

Superior vena caval obstruction

Superior vena caval (SVC) obstruction most commonly occurs as a result of extrinsic compression by a malignant bronchial tumour at the apex of the right lung. Although it is an uncomfortable condition, SVC obstruction is not itself life-threatening. The priority of acute management is therefore to relieve symptoms.

Causes

- Malignancy (accounts for 97% of cases):
  - lung cancer (80%)
  - lymphoma.
- Central venous catheters.
- Thrombosis.

Clinical features

The patient may complain of swelling of the face, neck, arms and chest which is most pronounced first thing in the morning. In addition, headache, lethargy, weight loss and a cough may occur. Examination may reveal the following:

- oedema of the face, neck and arms
- plethora of the face
- distended superficial veins of the neck and upper chest
- signs of lung cancer itself, such as apical dullness, reduced air entry or a pleural effusion
- lymphadenopathy (solid tumours or lymphoma).

Management

The priority of acute management is to relieve symptoms and diagnose the underlying pathology of obstruction.

- Sit the patient upright. This helps to relieve oedema of the face, neck and arms.
- Commence oxygen via a mask.
- Give simple analgesia to reduce discomfort.
- Remove the central venous catheter, if present, as this may be causing the SVC obstruction.

- Take a chest X-ray (antero-posterior and lateral view) to look for evidence of a right apical lung mass. A CT scan of the chest with contrast should be performed subsequently.
- Send a sputum sample for cytology to look for malignant cells.
- Discuss the case with the on-call oncologist for further advice on management.
- Steroids (oral dexamethasone) are beneficial in reducing the swelling of tissue associated with malignancy, and therefore help to relieve SVC obstruction. However, because they alter the histology of lymphomatous tissue, steroids should generally only be commenced once the tissue diagnosis has been made.
- A tissue diagnosis may be made by bronchoscopy or CT-guided biopsy.
- Further treatment may consist of radiotherapy (for non-small-cell bronchial carcinoma) or chemotherapy (for small-cell bronchial carcinoma or lymphoma).
- If the symptoms of SVC obstruction are severe or the tumour is not responsive to radiotherapy or chemotherapy, stenting of the SVC under radiological guidance may be attempted.

Further reading

- Wudel LJ Jr and Nesbitt JC (2001) Superior vena cava syndrome. *Curr Treat Options Oncol.* **2**: 77–91.

7 Abdominal conditions

Appendicitis

This is one of the commonest causes of acute abdominal pain, with a lifetime risk of 7%. In most cases, the appendicular lumen becomes obstructed by a faecalith and this causes the inflammation. Occasionally, especially in the elderly, a carcinoma of the caecum may cause the obstruction, and appendicitis is then the presenting feature of this more significant pathology.

Clinical features

The features of appendicitis are summarised in Table 16.

Table 16   Characteristics of the pain of appendicitis

Site	Starts centrally, and then moves to right iliac fossa (RIF)
Onset	Gradual over 2–3 days
Severity	Variable
Character	Initially vague but becomes more sharp
Progression	Constant
Duration	A few days
Precipitating factors	No specific factors
Relieving factors	Analgesia
Radiation	Central to RIF

The diagnosis of appendicitis is often extremely difficult, and various scoring systems have been developed. The only one of any clinical use is the modified Alvarado (or MANTREL) score.

- Migrating RIF pain (1 point).
- Anorexia (1 point).
- Nausea/vomiting (1 point).
- Tender RIF (2 points).

- Rebound tenderness (1 point).
- Elevated temperature > 37.5°C (1 point).
- Leukocytosis (1 point).

The higher the number of the above features that are present, the greater the likelihood is that the patient has acute appendicitis, with a score of ≥ 6 being considered diagnostic. Scores of ≤ 4 reliably exclude the diagnosis, but scores of 5–6 have poor reliability for either diagnosis or exclusion. These patients need careful and repeated clinical evaluation. Spontaneous improvement of symptoms strongly suggests that the patient does not have appendicitis, whereas worsening symptoms or signs warrant surgical exploration. Rovsing's sign (pain felt in the left iliac fossa during palpation of the RIF, due to peritoneal irritation) can be helpful, but has poor sensitivity and specificity.

Children, women and the elderly often present atypically and therefore require a higher index of suspicion. Again, repeated clinical evaluation over the period of an overnight hospital admission should be considered in all uncertain cases. Children should be distracted during clinical examination of their abdomen so that genuine signs are elicited.

Investigations

Apart from routine blood tests (e.g. FBC may show a raised white blood count and C-reactive protein), there is no consensus regarding the use of abdominal ultrasound or diagnostic laparoscopy.

Management

Some surgeons prefer to proceed directly to appendicectomy, while others perform laparoscopy to exclude gynaecological causes (e.g. acute salpingitis) in female patients, and then proceed to laparoscopic appendicectomy if the appendix appears to be inflamed. Some centres perform all of their appendicectomies using a laparoscopic approach. There is no compelling evidence to suggest that there is any significant difference in outcome between open and laparoscopic approaches. The main point is that it is important to try to perform the appendicectomy before the appendix perforates, otherwise the operation will be more difficult and there will be an increased risk of post-operative sepsis. Antibiotic cover with cefotaxime plus metronidazole is usually instituted peri-operatively, although local practices vary with regard to the length of treatment required.

Further reading

- Anderson RE (2004) Meta-analysis of the clinical and laboratory diagnosis of appendicitis. *Br J Surg.* **91**: 28–37.
- Ohmana C, Yang O and Frank C (1995) Diagnostic scores for acute appendicitis – Abdominal Pain Diagnostic Group. *Eur J Surg.* **161**: 273–81.
- Sooriakumaran P, Lovell DP and Brown R (2005) A comparison of clinical judgement of Accident and Emergency doctors and the modified Alvarado Score in evaluating the need for surgical referral in cases of suspected acute appendicitis. *Int J Surg.* **3**: 49–52.

Acute pancreatitis

Aetiology

Acute pancreatitis is an acute inflammation of the pancreas caused by activated pancreatic enzymes (e.g. trypsin, chymotrypsin) leaking into the substance of the pancreas. Obstruction of the main pancreatic duct of Wirsung (e.g. by a gallstone) can cause this. Other causes (with a helpful acronym) include the following.

- Gallstones.
- Ethanol.
- Trauma.
- Steroids.
- Mumps and other viruses.
- Autoimmune diseases (e.g. polyarteritis nodosa).
- Scorpion bites.
- Hyperlipidaemia.
- ERCP.
- Drugs (e.g. oestrogen-containing OCP, azathioprine, thiazide diuretics).

Gallstones and alcohol account for over 80% of cases of acute pancreatitis.

Clinical features

Table 17 Characteristics of the pain of acute pancreatitis

Site	Epigastric
Onset	Sudden
Severity	Variable, from very mild to severe and necrotising
Character	Typically gnawing, but variable
Progression	Worsens gradually
Duration	Variable
Precipitating factors	Often an alcoholic binge
Relieving factors	Opiate analgesia
Radiation	Through to the back

The patient may be distressed, sweating and mildly pyrexial. They may feel nauseated or vomit. Signs of shock requiring immediate resuscitation may be present due to fluid sequestration into the retroperitoneal and peritoneal spaces. The abdomen is often very tender in the epigastrium, and this sign may be accompanied by voluntary guarding (remember that this is a sign of pain and not peritonitis, in which involuntary guarding may occur). Grey–Turner's and Cullen's signs (bluish discoloration in the flanks and periumbilical areas, respectively) are found in haemorrhagic pancreatitis, with spread of blood retroperitoneally to these areas. Therefore they only occur in a minority of cases and they take several days to develop.

A serum amylase level greater than ten times the upper limit of normal is considered pathognomonic of pancreatitis. Levels greater than three times the upper limit of normal are usually due to pancreatitis. Smaller increases in serum amylase levels may be found in many other conditions that cause an acute abdomen (e.g. peptic ulcer disease, cholecystitis, bowel infarction, peritonitis). Serum lipase concentrations remain higher for longer than serum amylase levels, and are more specific to the pancreas, so can be used for equivocal cases.

Assessment

Severity is assessed using the Ranson criteria (*see* Table 18).

Table 18   Ranson criteria

At admission	During first 48 hours
Age > 55 years	Haematocrit decreases by > 10%
WBC > 16 × 10⁹/litre	Blood urea increases by > 2 mmol/litre
Fasting blood glucose > 11 mmol/litre	Serum calcium < 2 mmol/litre
Serum LDH > 350 IU/litre (double normal)	PaO_2 < 8 kPa
Serum AST > 60 U/litre (six times normal)	Base excess > −4 mmol/litre (base deficit > 4 mmol/litre) Estimated fluid sequestration > 6 litres

Patients who meet less than three of these criteria have a mortality of less than 1%, and those who meet more than six criteria have a mortality of 90%. Other scoring systems such as the Imrie and the APACHE II (Applied Physiology and Chronic Health Evaluation II) are also used in some centres, but are broadly similar to the Ranson system.

Investigations

These are performed according to the Ranson criteria. In addition, the following are required:

- serum amylase (and/or serum lipase)
- U&Es (a raised urea:creatinine ratio suggests dehydration, possibly due to fluid sequestration)
- LFTs (raised bilirubin levels may be found if the inflammation obstructs biliary drainage)
- clotting profile (DIC is a complication of acute pancreatitis)
- chest X-ray (small pleural effusions may be seen)
- abdominal X-ray (absent psoas shadows and a sentinel bowel loop adjacent to the pancreas due to local ileus may be seen)
- ECG (diminished T-waves may be seen)
- contrast-enhanced CT scan (this can make the diagnosis and demonstrate any necrosis present, as well as detecting complications such as abscesses and pseudocysts)
- ultrasound scan (not as good as CT for definition of the gland, but useful for demonstrating gallstones as the cause).

Management

This can range from simple resting of the gastrointestinal tract (nasogastric tube, NBM, IV fluids – 'drip and suck') to ITU management, depending on the severity of the disease. Surgery is generally reserved for haemorrhagic, necrotising pancreatitis ('necrosectomy') and for draining complications such as pseudocysts and abscesses. Medical management should consider the following:

- high-flow oxygen
- IV access and IV fluids
- IV analgesia (e.g. morphine titrated according to response)
- anti-emesis (e.g. cyclizine 50 mg IV)
- nasogastric tube
- nil by mouth; longer-term feeding should be with either total parenteral nutrition (TPN) or jejunal feeds in order to minimise pancreatic secretions
- urinary catheterisation for accurate monitoring of fluid balance (a CVP line may also be needed in more severe cases)
- transfer the patient to the HDU or ITU if three or more of Ranson's criteria are present

- antibiotics should not be used routinely, and abscesses should be drained
- ERCP and sphincterotomy decrease morbidity in cases of gallstone pancreatitis if performed within the first 72 hours after presentation
- somatostatin analogues (e.g. octreotide) have been used to suppress pancreatic secretions, although trials show conflicting results with regard to mortality reduction.

Further reading

- Santamaria JD (2002) Acute pancreatitis. In: TE Oh (ed.) *Intensive Care Manual* (4e). Butterworth Heinemann, Edinburgh.
- Raftery AT (2001) *Churchill's Pocketbook of Surgery* (2e). Churchill Livingstone, Edinburgh.
- Ranson JH, Rifkind KM, Roses DF *et al.* (1974) Prognostic signs and the role of operative management in acute pancreatitis. *Surg Gynecol Obstet.* **139:** 69–81.
- Neoptolemos JP, Carr-Locke DL, London NJ *et al.* (1988) Controlled trial of urgent endoscopic retrograde cholangiopancreatography and endoscopic sphincterotomy versus conservative treatment for acute pancreatitis due to gallstones. *The Lancet.* **2:** 979–83.

Ascending cholangitis

Infection in the common bile duct (CBD) can be fatal if it is not treated promptly. It presents with jaundice, epigastric pain, and rigors caused by high intermittent fever (Charcot's triad). The patient will therefore present with raised inflammatory markers (e.g. white blood count, C-reactive protein) and signs of septicaemia (*see* p. 253). Elderly patients may sometimes present with collapse or septicaemia with little or no jaundice, making the diagnosis more difficult in these cases. Cholangitis spreads up the CBD – hence the term 'ascending'. It can therefore give rise to intrahepatic abscesses, which may rupture through the capsule of the liver and form intraperitoneal collections, causing peritonitis (*see* p. 107). Multiple small liver abscesses may also result from the suppurative process, and these may require percutaneous drainage (using CT guidance) or open drainage.

Cholangitis is caused by obstruction of the CBD, which is commonly benign (gallstones account for the majority of cases) and rarely malignant (strictures can result from carcinoma of the ampulla of Vater or head of pancreas). As a result, the CBD proximal to the site of obstruction will be dilated (> 7 mm in diameter), and this can be visualised on ultrasound scan, as can any obstructing gallstone. Cholangitis can also occur as a complication of biliary tract surgery or intervention, and is seen in more than 1% of cases after percutaneous transhepatic cholangiography (PTC).

The aerobic and anaerobic flora of the bowel (e.g. *E. coli*, *Streptococcus faecalis*, *Klebsiella*, *Bacteroides*) are the typical pathogenic organisms, and therefore antibiotic cover is with a third-generation cephalosporin such as cefotaxime, plus metronidazole. However, the basic principle that antibiotics do not treat pus applies here. Therefore drainage of pus is also necessary, and this is usually accomplished via an endoscopic sphincterotomy, which also allows extraction of any obstructing gallstone. If this fails, conventional open surgical drainage is performed. As is true of all surgical emergencies, appropriate fluid resuscitation is imperative.

If the sepsis becomes systemic, renal failure can result, with ensuing septic shock, multi-organ dysfunction syndrome (MODS) and multi-organ failure (MOF) (*see* p. 255). The mortality rate in these patients is very high.

Further reading

- Hanau LH and Steigbigel NH (2004) Acute (ascending) cholangitis. *Infect Dis Clin North Am.* **14:** 521–46.
- Muir CA (2004) Acute ascending cholangitis. *Clin J Oncol Nurs.* **8:** 157–60.

Acute peritonitis

Acute peritonitis is an acute inflammation of the peritoneum. It may be local or generalised, and bacterial or aseptic. Localised peritonitis is due to transmural inflammation of a viscus (e.g. appendicitis, cholecystitis, diverticulitis). In its role as the 'abdominal policeman', the omentum may wrap around the inflammation and keep it localised. However, if the viscus perforates or the omentum does not wrap around adequately, generalised peritonitis with inflammation of the entire peritoneum will result. Aseptic peritonitis results from the presence of bile, blood, urine, pancreatic or gastric secretions in the peritoneum, which causes irritation and subsequent inflammation. This can become secondarily infected, leading to bacterial peritonitis.

Causes

Table 19   Causes of acute peritonitis

Bacterial peritonitis	*Aseptic peritonitis*
From the outside: penetrating abdominal trauma; post-laparotomy infection; chronic ambulatory peritoneal dialysis	*Bile:* damage to the gall bladder or its ducts from iatrogenic injury after a biliary tract operation, PTC or liver biopsy (the gall bladder very rarely perforates after acute cholecystitis because of its dual blood supply from the liver bed as well as the cystic artery)
From intra-abdominal viscera: gangrene or perforation of appendix, gall bladder, diverticulum or peptic ulcer; bowel infarction; post-operative intestinal suture dehiscence	*Blood:* e.g. ruptured spleen after intra-abdominal trauma
From the bloodstream: as part of a septicaemia (typically streptococcal or pneumococcal)	*Urine:* e.g. intraperitoneal rupture of the bladder from trauma or as a complication of transurethral resection of bladder tumour when tumour is on anterior surface of bladder
From the female genital tract: acute salpingitis	*Pancreas:* e.g. acute pancreatitis
From aseptic causes that become secondarily infected	*Stomach:* e.g. perforated gastric ulcer (much less common than perforated duodenal ulcer)

Clinical features

Sudden onset of extreme pain, aggravated by coughing and movement (as this causes the two layers of the inflamed peritoneum to rub together).

- Fever.
- Nausea and vomiting.
- Abdominal tenderness (may start in one quadrant and progress to involve the whole abdomen as localised peritonitis becomes generalised).
- Involuntary guarding, board-like rigidity and rebound tenderness are classic signs of peritonitis.
- Abdominal distension.
- Absent bowel sounds (once an ileus supervenes).
- Patient looks very ill.
- Rapid, shallow breathing (to compensate the metabolic acidosis that results from peritonitis).
- Hypotensive shock is a late sign (due to massive fluid sequestration into the peritoneum).
- Septicaemia (typically Gram-negative) can occur if the cause is infective.
- Air under the diaphragm is seen on erect chest X-ray in many but not all cases.

Investigations

- FBC (white blood count will usually be raised).
- U&Es (a raised urea:creatinine ratio may be found due to dehydration or due to acute renal failure as a complication of peritonitis).
- Serum amylase or lipase (to diagnose pancreatitis).
- Clotting profile (DIC is a complication of peritonitis).
- Group and save or cross-match (in case blood is required for surgery).
- Chest X-ray (to detect air under the diaphragm).
- Abdominal X-ray (distended bowel with ileus and sentinel loop with pancreatitis may be seen).
- ECG (to confirm the patient's fitness for surgery if required, and to monitor for cardiac complications such as myocardial infarction).
- CT scan (for diagnosis, especially if pancreatitis is suspected).
- Ultrasound scan (to look for free fluid and localised collections).

Management

As with all life-threatening emergencies, ABC is the priority. High-flow oxygen is always imperative. Pain relief with IV opiates and IV fluid resuscitation (titrated according to electrolyte imbalances) are priorities. The bowel should be rested by nasogastric tube decompression and keeping the patient nil by mouth. Adequate monitoring of fluid status requires urinary catheterisation (and a CVP line in more severe cases). Broad-spectrum antibiotics to cover both aerobic and anaerobic faecal flora (e.g. a third-generation cephalosporin such as cefotaxime together with metronidazole) should be used.

Except in cases of acute pancreatitis (*see* p. 102), surgical exploration after resuscitation is required in the vast majority of cases. Only in a few cases of perforated duodenal ulcer in which the perforation appears contained and the patient is deemed unfit for surgery is conservative management alone attempted. Operative management involves an exploratory laparotomy, usually via a full midline incision. During surgery, thorough debridement and lavage should be performed and the underlying cause dealt with. A stoma may be preferable to anastomosis, and drains should be considered.

Death occurs in 40% of cases of generalised peritonitis, and time to theatre as well as peri-operative fluid and electrolyte management are crucial. A CVP line only measures right atrial pressure, and is thus an often inaccurate surrogate for the pressure within the left heart and systemic circulation. Therefore severe cases may require the insertion of a Swann–Ganz (pulmonary artery) catheter to measure the left-sided ('wedge') pressure.

Further reading

- Ellis H, Calne R and Watson C (1998) *Lecture Notes in General Surgery* (9e). Blackwell Science, Oxford.
- Marshall JC (2004) Intra-abdominal infections. *Microbes Infect.* 6: 1015–25.
- Colizza S and Rossi S (2001) Antibiotic prophylaxis and treatment of surgical abdominal sepsis. *J Chemother.* 1: 193–201.

Liver failure

The liver excretes waste products, produces proteins (including albumin and clotting factors), and is essential for the metabolism of carbohydrates and lipids to produce energy. Liver failure therefore leads to a wide range of clinical manifestations that stem from impairment of its functions.

Aetiology

Liver failure may occur either in previously fit individuals (acute liver failure) or in individuals with chronic liver disease.

Acute liver failure

The main causes are as follows:

- drugs (e.g. paracetamol)
- viral hepatitis (e.g. hepatitis A and B)
- biliary obstruction (e.g. gallstones).

Liver failure associated with chronic liver disease

The main causes are as follows:

- alcohol
- viral hepatitis (e.g. hepatitis B and C)
- chronic biliary obstruction (e.g. primary biliary cirrhosis, carcinoma of head of pancreas)
- other rarer causes (e.g. haemochromatosis, Wilson's disease, α_1-antitrypsin deficiency, autoimmune hepatitis).

Clinical features

Look for the following evidence of liver failure itself:

- jaundice
- confusion or drowsiness (due to hepatic encephalopathy)
- liver flap (asterixis) (due to hepatic encephalopathy)
- bleeding tendency
- hypoglycaemia
- oliguria (due to hepatorenal syndrome).

The following should only be present if there is established chronic liver disease:

● clubbing
● Dupuytren's contracture
● palmar erythema
● spider naevi
● gynaecomastia
● hepatomegaly.

Patients may develop portal hypertension as a result of cirrhosis associated with chronic liver disease. This gives rise to features such as ascites, oesophageal varices (which may bleed) and caput medusae.

Management

● Assess the grade of encephalopathy using the scale shown in Table 20. In addition, any patient with a Glasgow Coma Scale score of ≤ 8 requires intubation, as they cannot protect their airway.

Table 20   Grading system for hepatic encephalopathy

Grade of hepatic encephalopathy	Clinical description
1	Drowsy but coherent, change in mood
2	Drowsy, confused
3	Very drowsy but rousable
4	Comatose, barely rousable

● Send blood samples urgently for:
  – U&Es (look for hypokalaemia or evidence of hepatorenal syndrome)
  – LFTs:
    (i) ↑ alkaline phosphatase (ALP) > ↑ transaminases suggests biliary obstruction
    (ii) ↑ transaminases > ↑ ALP suggests liver parenchymal damage
  – gamma-glutamyl transferase (GGT)
  – glucose (look for hypoglycaemia)
  – paracetamol level
  – FBC
  – clotting profile (PT may be prolonged).

- Prevention and treatment of hepatic encephalopathy:
  - a low protein diet is given to reduce nitrogen toxin production
  - regular lactulose is given and metabolised by colonic bacteria, thereby decreasing the colonic pH. The amount of ammonia produced by these bacteria is therefore reduced
  - neomycin is an antibiotic used as an alternative to lactulose in cases where diarrhoea is a problem.
- Order an ultrasound examination of the biliary tract to diagnose biliary obstruction, and if necessary discuss the options for biliary drainage with the surgical team.
- If there is evidence of bleeding, give vitamin K 10 mg IV and discuss the administration of blood products such as fresh frozen plasma (FFP) and platelets with the haematologist.
- If the patient is hypotensive or has renal impairment, insert a catheter, monitor urine output and consider central venous pressure (CVP) measurement. Hypotension is best treated with human albumin solution.
- Avoid the use of normal saline in these patients, as it may aggravate the presence of any ascites.
- Avoid the use of sedatives such as opioids or benzodiazepines. However, haloperidol may be useful if agitation occurs.
- Check blood sugar levels regularly with glucose stix, and give 10–50 ml 50% glucose intravenously as required to maintain normoglycaemia.
- It is extremely important to discuss cases at the earliest opportunity with a specialist liver unit for assessment of the need for transplantation. Table 21 lists the main indications for liver transplantation.

Table 21 King's College Hospital criteria for liver transplantation in acute liver failure

Four sets of criteria for liver transplantation

1 EITHER	Paracetamol overdose (OD) with:	Admission pH < 7.3
2 OR	Paracetamol OD with all three of:	PT > 100 seconds creatinine > 300 μmol/litre Grade 3–4 encephalopathy
3 OR	Non-paracetamol OD with:	PT > 100 seconds
4 OR	Non-paracetamol OD with any three of:	PT > 50 seconds Jaundice-to-encephalopathy interval > 7 days Age < 10 years or > 40 years Bilirubin > 300 μmol/litre Unfavourable aetiology: not drug-induced, not hepatitis A or B

Further reading

- Devlin J and O'Grady J (2000) *Indications for Referral and Assessment in Adult Liver Transplantation: a clinical guideline.* British Society of Gastroenterology, London; www.bsg.org.uk/clinical_prac/guidelines/adult_liver.htm

Large bowel obstruction

The line of demarcation between large bowel and small bowel is at the ileocaecal valve. Large bowel obstruction is typically caused by colorectal carcinoma (usually left-sided constricting tumours), diverticular disease, volvulus (sigmoid is more common than caecal) or toxic megacolon (due to ulcerative colitis). There are four cardinal signs and symptoms of bowel obstruction:

1   colicky abdominal pain
2   abdominal distension
3   absolute constipation (i.e. no faeces or flatus passed)
4   vomiting.

If the obstruction is higher up the gastrointestinal tract (i.e. in the small bowel), there are comparatively fewer small bowel loops proximal to the obstruction that will be distended, and therefore the abdominal distension will be slight. In addition, the proximal contents may be ejected from the mouth, making vomiting a prominent feature of small bowel obstruction. However, with large bowel obstruction there are many loops of bowel proximal to the obstruction that will be distended, causing significant abdominal distension and bloating. The distal loops are collapsed, so there is absolute constipation rather than vomiting. The distal collapse means that the rectum is empty on digital rectal examination. There will be colicky abdominal pain in both small and large bowel obstruction due to the peristalsing proximal bowel segment trying to push faeculent/faecal contents beyond the obstruction. This also causes tympanitic bowel sounds on auscultation. If the abdominal pain becomes severe and constant, this is a sign of impending bowel infarction and necessitates an urgent laparotomy.

An abdominal X-ray will show distended, peripherally placed bowel loops (said to look like a picture frame) with haustrations that go all the way across the bowel. An erect film will confirm air/fluid levels, although usually the supine film is sufficient to make the diagnosis. The differential diagnosis of pseudo-obstruction can usually be excluded on the basis of the history, the lack of bowel sounds and the digital rectal examination. However, the diagnosis can be confirmed with an instant enema.

It is important to look for distended small bowel on the abdominal X-ray. This will appear as distended centrally placed loops with valvulae coniventes that go only partly across the bowel. If these are present, this means that the ileocaecal valve is incompetent (80% of cases) and therefore the proximal dilation has progressed to the small bowel. However, if there are no dilated small bowel loops, this means that the ileocaecal valve is competent (20% of cases) and thus the dilation is limited by this competence. Therefore in these cases the caecum will become progressively more dilated until it perforates. A caecal diameter of > 10 cm on abdominal X-ray is a sign of imminent rupture, and urgent decompression is required.

An abdominal X-ray may also show the 'coffee-bean' appearance of distended bowel arising out of the left side of the pelvis (or occasionally the right side when this indicates a caecal volvulus). A barium enema may be helpful in doubtful cases, but should be replaced by a Gastrografin enema in cases of large bowel obstruction in case the contrast exudes into the peritoneum with a perforation. A Gastrografin enema will also show the stricture causing large bowel obstruction due to diverticular disease, and may show the 'apple-core' lesion of a colorectal carcinoma.

In toxic megacolon the patient is pyrexial, tachycardic, and has severe abdominal pain and tenderness, indicating impending bowel infarction. Abdominal X-ray shows dilatation of the transverse colon to > 5.5 cm, loss of haustrations (resulting in a 'lead-pipe' appearance), irregularity of the bowel wall contour, and pseudopolyps projecting into the dilated bowel segment. The patient will need a laparotomy with resection, high-dose steroids and antibiotic cover.

A sigmoidoscopy will identify any rectosigmoid tumours and allow decompression of a volvulus with a rectal flatus tube, which should be left *in situ* for 48 hours. An elective resection of the volved sigmoid can be performed at a later date if the patient is fit for surgery. If decompression is unsuccessful, or if there are signs of gangrene or perforation, laparotomy with resection of the volved segment is performed, and the two ends are brought out as a double-barrelled (Paul–Mickulicz) colostomy, which can be closed later.

With the exception of a volvulus that responds to flatus tube decompression, fit patients should always have an immediate laparotomy with antibiotic cover (typically a third-generation cephalosporin such as cefotaxime, plus metronidazole). The patient should be kept nil by mouth, have a nasogastric tube inserted to decompress the bowel, be given opiate analgesia, and be resuscitated with IV fluids tailored to their urine output, heart rate and pulse. It is important to cover both the patient's fluid maintenance requirements (3 litres per 24 hours in a 70 kg adult) and their fluid losses through sequestration in the bowel (up to 6 litres per 24 hours).

Stricturing diverticular disease causing large bowel obstruction requires resection of the lesion, closure of the distal stump, and formation of a colostomy using the proximal stump (Hartmann's operation). However, as over 65% of patients never have their Hartmann colostomy reversed, an alternative is to make a primary anastomosis and protect it with a proximal defunctioning colostomy, which can be more easily reversed at a later date.

An obstructing colorectal carcinoma requires a laparotomy with re-section of the lesion. Left-sided lesions usually require a left hemicolectomy and proximal defunctioning colostomy, and right-sided lesions require a right hemicolectomy. If the lesion is close to the rectum and therefore no anastomosis can be made, a Hartmann's operation can be performed.

Some experienced surgeons do not always perform a defunctioning colostomy in cases of large bowel obstruction, and perform on-table lavage to protect a primary anastomosis. This is never appropriate if there is perforation and contamination of the operative field. In patients who are unfit for operative management because they are too toxaemic at the time, the caecum can be decompressed with a caecostomy and the patient operated on after improvement (this is only necessary if the ileocaecal valve is competent).

Further reading

- Ellis H, Calne R and Watson C (1998) *Lecture Notes in General Surgery* (9e). Blackwell Science, Oxford.
- Raftery AT (2001) *Churchill's Pocketbook of Surgery* (2e). Churchill Livingstone, Edinburgh.

Small bowel obstruction

The clinical features of small bowel obstruction are discussed in the section on large bowel obstruction (*see* p. 114), which should be read first. A high obstruction will present with early bilious vomiting, whereas a lower obstruction is likely to present with later faeculent vomiting. The two main causes of small bowel obstruction are adhesions and hernias. Occasionally, Crohn's disease and gallstone ileus may be causative factors. Very rarely, small bowel obstruction may be caused by a jejunal or duodenal tumour.

Pyrexia, tachycardia, continuous pain and localised tenderness suggest impending strangulation of bowel. Examination of the hernial orifices should identify a strangulated hernia (*see* p. 119). Adhesions are caused by loops of bowel sticking together after the fibrotic response to previous surgery. Therefore the management of adhesive small bowel obstruction is conservative, as surgery to remove adhesions is usually counter-productive. A history of previous surgery, normal hernial examination and an abdominal scar therefore suggest adhesions as the cause. The patient should be kept nil by mouth, have a nasogastric tube inserted, be given IV fluids, and be monitored regularly. If there are signs of a strangulated hernia or impending bowel strangulation, a laparotomy should be performed and non-viable bowel resected with on-table lavage and primary anastomosis. Non-viable bowel is identified by:

- absence of peristalsis
- loss of sheen
- loss of pulsation in the mesentery
- black discoloration (if there is plum discoloration, it may respond to wrapping in warm saline-soaked packs for a few minutes).

Further reading

- Ellis H, Calne R and Watson C (1998) *Lecture Notes in General Surgery* (9e). Blackwell Science, Oxford.
- Raftery AT (2001) *Churchill's Pocketbook of Surgery* (2e). Churchill Livingstone, Edinburgh.

Mesenteric ischaemia and infarction

Just as the coronary vessels and the carotid arteries are affected by athero-sclerotic disease, so are the mesenteric arteries. Thus patients with mesenteric atherosclerosis will have the same risk factors as those with ischaemic heart disease, cerebrovascular disease and peripheral vascular disease – that is, male sex, older age, smoking, diabetes, hypertension and hypercholesterolaemia. Mesenteric 'angina' occurs when the blood flow to the bowel is impaired, so is manifested as abdominal pain after eating. As with the coronary, carotid and peripheral limb arteries, acute occlu-sion can occur on top of this background chronic atheromatous disease, causing infarction of the supplied bowel. The bowel will bleed, resulting in bleeding per rectum which may be so severe that blood transfusion is required.

Mesenteric infarction can also result from an embolus lodging in the mesenteric circulation from the left atrium in patients with atrial fibril-lation, a mural thrombus post-MI, a vegetation on an endocarditic heart valve, or an atheromatous plaque on the aorta. Less commonly, occlusion can result from aortic dissection. Venous occlusion will also result in bowel infarction, and will in addition cause portal hypertension and its features (see p. 111). Both arterial and venous mesenteric occlusion may also be caused by the oral contraceptive pill and thrombophilia.

The patient with bowel infarction will be in severe pain, toxaemic, and require an urgent laparotomy to resect the gangrenous and perforated bowel. A mesenteric angiogram will identify the extent of infarction prior to surgery. Even with surgery and the peri-operative measures common to most general surgical emergencies (nil by mouth, IV fluids, analgesia, antibiotics, etc.), the prognosis is poor. This is because most of these patients are old and infirm with extensive disease and significant cardio-vascular comorbidity.

Further reading

- Ellis H, Calne R and Watson C (1998) *Lecture Notes in General Surgery* (9e). Blackwell Science, Oxford.
- Ottinger LW (2002) Mesenteric arteries. In: PJ Morris and RA Malt (eds) *Oxford Textbook of Surgery*. Oxford University Press, Oxford.

Strangulated hernia

A hernia is the protrusion of a viscus (organ) through its normal coverings to an ectopic site. The commonest hernias are abdominal. The abdominal contents protrude through their peritoneal coverings due to weaknesses in the abdominal wall.

The classic features of a hernia on examination are as follows.

- Reducible lump – this refers to the fact that the hernia can be pushed back into the abdominal cavity. However, not all hernias are reducible.
- Cough impulse – the thrill felt by the palpating fingers when the patient coughs. Palpating a cough impulse becomes difficult in large hernias with tight necks.

There is much confusion about the terms 'irreducible', 'incarcerated' and 'strangulated', not least because surgeons often use such terms indiscriminately.

- An *irreducible* hernia cannot be reduced, and is therefore 'stuck', usually due to adhesions of its contents to the inner wall of the peritoneal sac.
- An *incarcerated* hernia is irreducible but not strangulated. However, because some clinicians equate it to a strangulated hernia, this term is best avoided.
- A *strangulated* hernia has a tight neck cutting off the blood supply to the contents. Unless relieved, the bowel contained within the hernia will become gangrenous and die, resulting in perforation and peritonitis. Hernias with tight necks (e.g. femoral hernias) are more likely to strangulate than those with wide necks (e.g. incisional or inguinal hernias).

The risk of strangulation means that asymptomatic femoral hernias should be surgically repaired electively within 1 month, and symptomatic femoral hernias should be repaired on the next available operating list. When a hernia progresses from being simply irreducible to being strangulated, the patient will become systemically unwell and show signs and symptoms of small bowel obstruction (*see* p. 114 and p. 117). A strangulated femoral hernia will typically occur in elderly female patients (due to their tighter femoral rings), and on examination a hard lump can be felt in the region of the femoral canal (below and lateral to the pubic tubercle). Due to the strangulation, the typical features of reducibility and cough impulse will not be present. The patient must be kept nil by mouth, given IV fluids, antibiotics and analgesia, and undergo urgent surgery using a high extra-peritoneal incision (McEvedy approach) to facilitate decompression of the hernial sac and resection of any non-viable bowel (*see* p. 117).

Occasionally, only omentum and not bowel is strangulated, and therefore the patient does not appear as unwell and is at much lower risk of peritonitis. However, it is a brave clinician who does not assume bowel involvement in strangulated abdominal hernias, as the consequences of error are potentially life-threatening.

Further reading

- Smith CP and Hernon C (eds) (2000) *MRCS System Modules: essential revision notes*. Pastest, Knutsford.
- Ellis H, Calne R and Watson C (1998) *Lecture Notes in General Surgery* (9e). Blackwell Science, Oxford.

Upper gastrointestinal bleeding

An upper gastrointestinal bleed may present with haematemesis or melaena. It is associated with a significant mortality, and must be managed as a top priority whether in Accident and Emergency or on the ward.

Aetiology

- Gastric ulceration (35–50% of upper gastrointestinal bleeds) or duodenal ulceration.
- Gastritis or duodenitis.
- Bleeding oesophageal varices associated with portal hypertension.
- Arterio-venous malformation.
- Mallory–Weiss tear (caused by excessive vomiting).
- Bleeding diatheses (e.g. warfarin usage).
- Meckel's diverticulum.

Clinical features

Look for a history of any underlying causes, such as peptic ulcer disease, liver disease or alcohol abuse. Pay attention to the drug history, particularly the use of NSAIDs and warfarin.

Features which suggest a significant upper gastrointestinal bleed include the following:

- witnessed blood loss (haematemesis or melaena) > 100 ml
- signs of shock (e.g. hypotension, postural blood pressure drop, tachycardia, cold extremities).

In addition, the patient may show signs of factors predisposing to upper gastrointestinal bleeding, such as liver failure or evidence of previous gastrointestinal surgery.

Management

Call senior colleagues for help the moment you suspect a significant upper gastrointestinal bleed. Then take the following steps immediately.

- Obtain IV access with two large cannulae (preferably brown).
- Keep the patient nil by mouth.

- Send blood urgently for:
  - FBC (note that Hb does not drop within 24 hours of an acute bleed)
  - clotting profile (impairment of PT occurs in liver failure and with warfarin usage)
  - cross-match at least 4 units of blood if the bleed is significant (*see* above); otherwise group and save blood for possible transfusion later
  - U&Es (urea is disproportionately raised compared with creatinine)
  - LFTs (abnormal results suggest a hepatic pathology which may promote bleeding via portal hypertension and impairment of clotting).
- If the bleed is significant, give a bolus of IV omeprazole 80 mg followed by an omeprazole infusion (8 mg per hour for 72 hours). However, if the index of suspicion for upper gastrointestinal bleeding is lower, give 40 mg IV omeprazole daily.
- Catheterise the patient and monitor their urine output.
- If there are signs of shock or oliguria, consider central venous access in order to monitor fluid status.
- An oesophago-gastro-duodenoscopy (OGD) must be performed to look for the source of bleeding, but the timing of this will depend on the severity of the bleed. A significant bleed should be discussed with the on-call endoscopist with a view to OGD within 12 hours. A less severe bleed may have OGD delayed for 24 to 48 hours.
- If clotting abnormalities or thrombocytopenia are present, speak to the on-call haematologist about correction with blood products (e.g. fresh frozen plasma, platelets) and/or vitamin K.

Management of oesophageal varices

Bleeding oesophageal varices may occur in portal hypertension associated with cirrhosis, most commonly due to alcohol abuse. If varices are suspected, call senior colleagues for help immediately, and correct clotting abnormalities (*see* above). An OGD should be performed as soon as possible, but if there is a delay in endoscopy, the registrar may consider one of the following.

- IV terlipressin (a vasopressin analogue) may be given to constrict the splanchnic circulation and reduce bleeding. Intravenous octreotide is a somatostatin analogue that also causes splanchnic vasoconstriction, but it is now rarely used.

- A Sengstaken–Blakemore tube may be used after terlipressin has been given in order to tamponade the stomach contents, but it should only be inserted by appropriately skilled individuals.

Further reading

- British Society of Gastroenterology Endoscopy Committee (2002) Non-variceal upper gastrointestinal haemorrhage: guidelines. *Gut.* **51 (Suppl. 4):** iv1–6.
- Jalan R and Hayes PC (2004) *UK Guidelines on the Management of Variceal Haemorrhage in Cirrhotic Patients.* British Society of Gastroenterology, London; www.bsg.org.uk/clinical_prac/guidelines

Lower gastrointestinal bleeding

Gastrointestinal haemorrhage may be from the upper or lower gastrointestinal tract, the demarcation being at the ligament of Treitz at the duodenojejunal junction. Upper gastrointestinal bleeding presents with haematemesis and melaena, whereas lower gastrointestinal bleeding presents with frank, red blood per rectum.

Management

- Lie the patient in a head-down position and use pressure as appropriate.
- Assess and replace the blood loss (*see* p. 121 and p. 250).
- Diagnose the cause.
- Treat and control the cause of the bleeding.

There may be a general cause of the bleeding (e.g. bleeding diathesis), or it may be specific to the gastrointestinal tract, as described below.

Investigation

Colonoscopy, angiography or a white-cell scan may be used to locate the source of lower gastrointestinal bleeding.

Angiodysplasia

Angiodysplasia is a condition characterised by mucosal or submucosal vascular malformations, most often in the caecum or ascending colon. Diagnosis is usually made by excluding other causes and confirmed by angiography. Colonoscopic diathermy or resection may be required, as this type of bleeding is usually from multiple abnormal vessels rather than having a single focus.

Diverticular disease

Diverticular disease is a condition in which the mucosa of the bowel (typically the sigmoid colon, descending colon and caecum) herniates through the muscle wall to give rise to multiple outpouchings termed diverticula. The latter are due to a chronic increase in intraluminal pressure causing the herniations, and are thus more common with increasing age and low-fibre diets that cause constipation.

Diverticular disease is the commonest cause of sudden, profuse, bright red bleeding per rectum in an elderly patient. It often requires open surgical management to ligate the bleeding vessel.

Haemorrhoids

Haemorrhoids are dilated rectal veins typically found at the 3, 7 and 11 o'clock positions around the anus. Bleeding from haemorrhoids ('piles') is rarely torrential, and is unlikely to require fluid resuscitation or surgical management in the acute setting. Direct pressure on the piles using a pad is usually enough to stop the bleeding.

Further reading

- Steele RJC (2000) Rectal bleeding and altered bowel habit. In: IMA Ledingham (ed.) *The RCSE SELECT Programme. Module 1.* Centre for Medical Education, University of Dundee, Dundee.
- Downs R (2001) Gastrointestinal haemorrhage. In: R Ashford and N Evans (eds) *Surgical Critical Care.* Greenwich Medical Media Ltd, London.

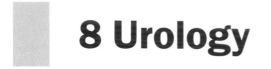

8 Urology

Testicular torsion

Testicular torsion is most common in the 12–18 years age group, but should be suspected in any young male patient presenting with acute abdominal or testicular pain (the testes originate embryologically in the abdomen, and therefore pain from the testes can be referred to the abdomen). The spermatic cord can twist in the scrotum of patients who have an incompletely descended testis, a high investment of the tunica vaginalis with a horizontally lying testis, or a long mesorchium.

The patient usually presents with a history of sudden onset of severe pain that occurs at rest or following straining, lifting, exercise or masturbation. Examination reveals a swollen, excruciatingly painful testis drawn up to the groin, often with a red, oedematous scrotum. If associated with pyrexia and leucocytosis in a sexually active male, the diagnosis is more commonly acute epididymo-orchitis, which will respond to antibiotic management. The problem is that it can be impossible to differentiate clinically between the two, in which case the management should be as for torsion. In addition, the cyst of Morgagni that lies at the peak of the epididymis can also twist (torsion of the cyst of Morgagni). Again a provisional diagnosis of testicular torsion should be made and the patient managed as for that condition.

A colour duplex ultrasound examination can differentiate between torsion and epididymo-orchitis (because with torsion the blood flow to the testis is reduced), but unless performed immediately this investigation will unnecessarily delay the time to definitive treatment, and should therefore be omitted. That is to say, the diagnosis is a clinical one and time to intervention is of paramount importance (as in the management of tension pneumothorax; see p. 40).

All patients with suspected testicular torsion should therefore be kept nil by mouth, have IV fluid hydration, and be taken to theatre within 1 hour of arrival in Accident and Emergency (testicular infarction and loss will occur after 6 hours of torsion). The testis should be explored, and if the diagnosis of torsion is confirmed, the testis should be untwisted and fixed to the scrotum to prevent future twisting. As the predisposing factors for torsion are congenital, the other testis is also likely to be susceptible to torsion and should therefore be fixed at the same operation. However, if after untwisting, the testis appears non-viable (i.e. infarcted), it should be surgically removed (orchidectomy) to prevent the development of sperm autoantibodies which will depress spermatogenesis in the remaining testis.

Further reading

- Dogra V and Bhatt S (2004) Acute painful scrotum. *Radiol Clin North Am*. **42**: 349–63.
- Cole FL and Vogler R (2004) The acute, non-traumatic scrotum: assessment, diagnosis and management. *J Am Acad Nurse Pract*. **16**: 50–6.

Ureteric colic

Ureteric colic (erroneously referred to as 'renal colic' by some) is a colicky abdominal pain extending from loin to groin (and sometimes testes) that typically occurs in young or middle-aged individuals (more commonly male). An important differential diagnosis that should always be considered is leaking/ruptured abdominal aortic aneurysm, and therefore a proper abdominal assessment including examination of the aorta is warranted.

Ureteric colic is caused by the presence of a calculus (stone) in the ureter, and is typically accompanied by urinary frequency, dysuria and microscopic haematuria (therefore urinalysis should be performed in suspected cases). If the stone is in the kidney or bladder, any resulting pain will not be colicky. Renal stones typically present with haematuria, infection or renal failure, whereas bladder calculi are more likely to cause pain at the tip of the penis during micturition. Renal stones can be managed conservatively or with a variety of procedures (e.g. extracorporeal shock-wave lithotripsy (ESWL), retrograde ureteroscopy or percutaneous nephrolithotomy). The management strategy that is chosen will depend on the size, location and physiological impact of the stone. Bladder stones can also be managed expectantly or removed endoscopically via cystoscopy.

Regardless of its location in the urinary tract, the stone is composed of a mixture of crystals within a protein matrix. The majority are composed of calcium in combination with oxalate (70–80%), phosphate (5–10%), struvite (magnesium ammonium phosphate – the so-called 'triple stone' that typically presents as a staghorn calculus in the kidney; 5–10%) or urate (3–5%), although they may rarely include amino acids (e.g. cysteine, xanthine) or drugs (e.g. indinavir, triamterine). There are many factors that predispose to solute precipitation in the urine, leading to stone formation:

- low fluid intake
- urinary tract abnormality (e.g. pelvi-ureteric junction (PUJ) obstruction)
- urinary tract infection
- foreign body
- hypercalcaemia (e.g. hyperparathyroidism)
- hyperuricaemia (e.g. gout)
- renal tubular dysfunction (e.g. renal tubular acidosis)
- inborn errors of metabolism (e.g. cysteinuria)
- diet (e.g. high oxalate consumption due to excessive tea drinking, high animal protein intake due to eating large amounts of red meat).

The diagnosis is made from a kidney, ureters and bladder (KUB) X-ray (the calculus is radio-opaque in 90% of cases) and confirmed with an intravenous urogram (IVU) (relative contraindications include asthma, seafood allergy, diabetic on metformin, poor renal function and advanced age, all of which increase the risk of contrast-induced anaphylaxis) or spiral CT scan. An IVU not only demonstrates a filling defect due to the stone itself, but also shows any impairment of drainage caused by proximal obstruction by the stone, and a spiral CT scan demonstrates the stone itself together with any proximal obstruction. Spiral CT scanning is becoming more widespread, although some institutions (and urologists) still prefer the IVU.

Obstruction is unlikely to result from small calculi (< 4 mm in diameter), which can therefore be managed conservatively with increased oral fluid intake (> 2 litres/day) and analgesia (typically with NSAIDs such as diclofenac). However, if a stone causes significant obstruction to drainage (i.e. contrast is still seen on a delayed film and/or renal dysfunction – as detected by elevated serum urea and creatinine levels – is present), the patient should be admitted under the care of the urological team for further management in addition to fluids and analgesia. Continued obstruction in the absence of sepsis can be dealt with operatively with a retrograde ureteroscopy and stone extraction or ESWL. However, if the patient becomes septic, relief of the infected, obstructed urinary system by means of a percutaneous nephrostomy under radiological guidance should be undertaken urgently.

As the risk of recurrence of urinary stones is around 50%, patients who suffer two or more attacks should be referred to a metabolic medicine specialist for investigation and subsequent prophylactic management.

Further reading

- Ghali AM, Elmalik EM, Ibrahim AI *et al.* (1998) Cost-effective emergency diagnosis plan for urinary stone patients presenting with ureteric colic. *Eur Urol.* **33**: 529–37.
- Smith RC and Coll DM (2000) Helical computed tomography in the diagnosis of ureteric colic. *BJU Int.* **86 (Suppl. 1)**: 33–41.
- Simon J, Roumeguere T, Vaessen C *et al.* (1997) Conservative management of ureteric stones. *Acta Urol Belg.* **65**: 7–9.

Acute retention of urine

Aetiology

Acute retention of urine has a long list of causes that should be remembered systematically:

Local causes

- In the urethral lumen/bladder neck – posterior urethral valves (in boys), tumours, stones, blood clots (e.g. post-transurethral resection surgery), meatal stenosis.
- In the urethral or bladder wall – urethral trauma, strictures, tumours.
- Outside the wall – benign prostatic hypertrophy (BPH), constipation, pelvic cancer, pregnant uterus.

General causes

- Post-operative.
- Neurogenic – spinal cord injuries and diseases (e.g. syphilitic tabes, tumours, multiple sclerosis, diabetic autonomic neuropathy).
- Drugs (e.g. anticholinergic drugs, antidepressants, alcohol).

However, by far the commonest cause is BPH (especially in post-operative patients), and therefore a digital rectal examination is mandatory. Patients should receive prompt analgesia and management, as they may be in agony as well as having post-renal failure caused by the back pressure of urinary tract obstruction (suggested by renal dysfunction on serum electrolytes and upper urinary tract dilatation on ultrasound scan). A urethral catheter should be passed (if this is not possible, an introducer-assisted or suprapubic catheterisation should be performed). It is vital to record the amount of urine drained, as this gives some indication of the likely cause and the need for later surgery.

Patients with BPH can be discharged with a catheter *in situ* and brought back a week or so later for a trial without catheter (TWOC). Alpha-blockers (e.g. tamsulosin) and/or 5-α-reductase inhibitors (e.g. finasteride) may be used to try to control their disease medically, but many patients who fail TWOC will need definitive prostatic reduction surgery, typically performed by transurethral resection of the prostate (TURP).

Patients in clot retention after urological surgery will need to have a three-way catheter inserted with continuous irrigation using saline, otherwise the blood will not drain out. General post-operative patients who do not have other predisposing conditions for acute retention of urine may spontaneously pass urine after simple measures such as standing up in a warm room, hearing the sound of running water, or bathing in warm water.

Less common causes of acute retention of urine, such as tumours, strictures and stones, can be managed with ultrasound scan and cysto-urethroscopy. Any neurological signs associated with acute retention of urine should prompt full neurological examinations and appropriate referral. Cauda equina syndrome can present with acute retention of urine and is a surgical emergency (*see* p. 145).

Further reading

- Thomas K, Chow K and Kirby RS (2004) Acute urinary retention: a review of the aetiology and management. *Prostate Cancer Prostatic Dis.* 7: 32–7.
- Alan MS (2004) The role of alpha-blockers in the management of acute urinary retention caused by benign prostatic obstruction. *Eur Urol.* 45: 325–32.

Acute pyelonephritis

Acute pyelonephritis is defined as the acute inflammation of the kidney and renal pelvis. It classically presents with sudden onset of loin pain associated with pyrexia and loin tenderness on examination. Nausea and vomiting are common. Around 75% of patients will present following a lower urinary tract infection, and the causative organisms are similar, namely *E. coli* (80% of cases), *Proteus*, *Klebsiella* and *Enterobacter*. A urinalysis will normally show red blood cells and pus cells prior to any culture results. Systemic features of infection are present, namely raised white cell count, C-reactive protein and ESR, and positive blood cultures, and the patient appears toxic and unwell. Renal function may be impaired, with raised urea and creatinine levels.

As all of the above features are similar to those found in patients with infected and obstructed urinary systems caused by stone disease (*see* p. 128), imaging is needed to differentiate between the diagnoses. An IVU and/or ultrasound scan will typically show renal enlargement, collecting system dilatation and lobar nephronia (focal renal enlargement mimicking an intra-renal mass), with no accompanying calculus. However, in acute pyelonephritis, both the IVU and the ultrasound scan are often normal, making this a predominantly clinical diagnosis.

Less severe attacks can be managed at home and do not require hospitalisation. The choice of antibiotic varies according to local policy, but co-amoxyclav, aminoglycosides (e.g. gentamicin) and quinolones (e.g. ciprofloxacin) are all appropriate and should be continued for 2 weeks (almost 50% of patients will relapse even after this prolonged course, but most of these will respond to a further 2-week course). Fluid rehydration (remember the third-space losses with sepsis; *see* p. 253) with oral or IV fluids should also be instituted. If symptoms persist beyond 3 days or the patient is very unwell (e.g. exhibiting features of septic shock), they should be admitted for IV antibiotics and fluids. The development of a perinephric or renal abscess requires radiological or surgical drainage (remember that antibiotics do not treat pus, regardless of what a physician might say!).

Further reading

- McRae SN and Dairiki Shortliffe LM (2000) Bacterial infections of the genitourinary tract. In: EA Tanagho and JW McAninch (eds) *Smith's General Urology* (15e). Lange, New York.

Priapism

Priapism is a prolonged, painful erection in the absence of sexual stimulation, which is not relieved by orgasm. The erection involves the corpus cavernosum but not the corpus spongiosum. If priapism is left untreated or treated late, thrombosis can result, with subsequent permanent impotence. Even with prompt treatment there is a high rate of recurrence.

Penile or perineal trauma can create an arterial–sinusoidal shunt within the corpus cavernosum, causing a high-flow (non-ischaemic) priapism. However, more commonly there is low-flow (ischaemic) priapism due to persistent cavernosal relaxation. Here the main causes are drugs, especially those injected into the corpus cavernosum to treat erectile dysfunction (e.g. prostaglandin E1, papaverine, phentolamine).

A good patient history should differentiate between high- and low-flow causes. In doubtful cases a colour duplex ultrasound examination and blood gas analysis of the penile blood can be performed. In high-flow cases, pudendal arteriography and embolisation are usually successful, although in some cases open ligation of the abnormal vessels is required. In low-flow cases, a butterfly needle should be inserted into the corpus cavernosum and blood aspirated (which can be sent for blood gas analysis to make the diagnosis) until the aspirate is bright red. If this fails, the corpus cavernosum can be injected with phenylephrine (an α-blocker to cause vasoconstriction) every 10–15 minutes until the erection subsides.

If all of the above conservative methods fail to relieve the erection, surgery to establish a shunt between the corpus cavernosum and either the glans penis, the corpus spongiosum or the saphenous vein is necessary.

Further reading

- Sadeghi-Najed H, Dogra V, Seftel AD and Mohamed MA (2004) Priapism. *Radiol Clin North Am.* **42**: 427–43.
- Vilke GM, Harrigan RA, Ufberg JW and Chan TC (2004) Emergency evaluation and treatment of priapism. *J Emerg Med.* **26**: 325–9.

9 Vascular conditions

Ruptured abdominal aortic aneurysm

An aneurysm is an abnormal dilatation of a vessel. The incidence of abdominal aortic aneurysms increases with age. The other main risk factors are hypertension, hyperlipidaemia, ischaemic heart disease and peripheral vascular disease. Smoking has also been implicated in the development of abdominal aortic aneurysm, because free radicals damage major blood vessels.

Patients with ruptured abdominal aortic aneurysm present with the following features:

- severe central abdominal pain
- hypovolaemic shock.

In any patient with the above features, or with features suggestive of ureteric colic, a ruptured abdominal aortic aneurysm should be suspected first, as this is a true surgical emergency. Ruptured abdominal aortic aneurysm has a mortality of more than 70%, which drops to around 50% if the patient survives until he or she reaches hospital. Immediate resuscitation with colloid should be instituted (*see* p. 250), and the patient should be taken to theatre immediately for open laparotomy (with a midline incision from the xiphisternum to the pubis) by an experienced general/vascular surgeon. Endovascular repair is not appropriate in the emergency setting. Surgery involves control of the haemorrhage with clamps followed by repair of the aneurysm.

Abdominal aortic aneurysm can also present with epigastric or back pain, signifying a leak or imminent rupture. Helical CT scanning and CT angiography allow better three-dimensional visualisation than conventional CT scanning and ultrasound examination, and should be performed immediately. If these patients are operated on early, the risks of subsequent hypovolaemic shock, cardiac arrest and multi-system organ failure, with their consequent morbidity and mortality, are much reduced.

Further reading

- Cates JR (1997) Abdominal aortic aneurysms: clinical diagnosis and management. *J Manipulative Physiol Ther.* **20:** 557–61.
- Cao P and De Rango P (1999) Abdominal aortic aneurysms: current management. *Cardiologia.* **44:** 711–17.

Aortic dissection

Aortic dissection consists of a breach in the aortic wall leading to the tracking of blood through the tunica media and thus the formation of a second, 'false' aortic lumen. Dissection is classified as either type A (involving the ascending aorta) or type B (involving only the descending aorta) (*see* Figure 13 opposite). In addition, branches of the aorta which exit in the region of the dissection may be occluded. Aortic dissection is a life-threatening condition associated with a mortality of approximately 1% per hour.

Predisposing factors
- Hypertension (the commonest risk factor).
- Atherosclerosis.
- Connective tissue disease (e.g. Marfan's syndrome).
- Fibromuscular dysplasia.
- Iatrogenic causes (e.g. aortic/coronary angiography).

Clinical features
The patient classically complains of sudden-onset, tearing central chest pain which radiates to the back, between the shoulder blades. Careful examination may reveal the following:

- hypertension
- asymmetry of the upper limb, carotid or femoral pulses
- weak femoral pulses
- aortic incompetence (e.g. early diastolic murmur, wide pulse pressure, water-hammer pulse)
- paraplegia (if the great radicular spinal artery (at level T10) is involved)
- acute abdomen due to mesenteric ischaemia (if coeliac or superior mesenteric arteries are involved)
- oliguria/anuria (if renal arteries are involved)
- acute lower limb ischaemia (if the femoral artery is involved)
- rupture of the dissected aorta causes acute hypotension and shock, and is usually fatal.

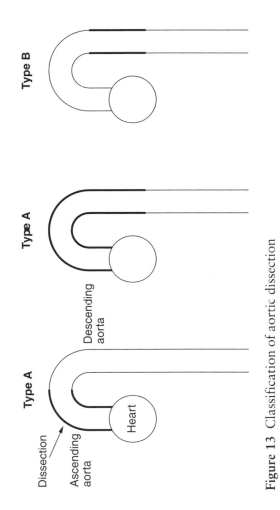

Figure 13 Classification of aortic dissection

Management

- Ensure that large-bore IV access is established, and that the patient is cross-matched, and has an urgent FBC with clotting profile.
- Various investigations may point to the diagnosis of aortic dissection:
  - a chest X-ray may show widening of the upper mediastinum, alteration of the aortic knuckle, or a left-sided pleural effusion
  - ECG may show left ventricular hypertrophy, indicating long-standing hypertension. Ischaemia or infarction may be evident if coronary artery involvement is present
  - the most commonly used method of diagnosing aortic dissection is either CT or MRI scanning (MRI is preferable). Aortic angiography may be used if these techniques are not available.
- Type A dissections must be treated surgically, as there is a high risk that they will extend proximally to cause aortic incompetence and heart failure. The on-call cardiothoracic surgeon must therefore be informed immediately.
- Type B dissections are treated medically by aggressive blood pressure control, commonly with sodium nitroprusside or labetolol.
- Closely monitor urine output, check U&Es and catheterise the patient as necessary.
- If mesenteric or acute limb ischaemia is suspected, urgent referral to the surgical team is necessary.

Acute limb ischaemia

Clinical features

Acute limb ischaemia is characterised by the six P's.

- Pain (becomes painless once the ischaemia is irreversible).
- Pallor.
- Pulselessness.
- Paraesthesiae (becomes anaesthesia with continuing ischaemia).
- Paralysis.
- Perishingly cold.

These features suggest a limb-threatening emergency and require prompt recognition and management. In the history, the patient may complain of a sudden onset of pain in the leg, which then becomes white and cold. In time, the other features of paraesthesiae (and then anaesthesia) and muscle paralysis develop due to continuing ischaemia. The commonest cause of an acutely ischaemic limb is embolism from atrial fibrillation, recent MI or aortic aneurysm. However, it can also be due to thrombosis in a known atherosclerotic patient (this is suggested if the patient shows features of chronic arterial disease, such as intermittent claudication, prolonged capillary refill, diminished Buerger's angle, decreased ankle:brachial pressure index, loss of pulses, venous guttering and ischaemic ulceration). Hair loss is said to be a sign of peripheral vascular disease, but is in reality a poor sign.

Examination of the pulses will give an indication of the site of blockage, which is most often in the superficial femoral artery. The longer the block is left, the less likely it is that any intervention will be successful, so it is crucial to begin heparinisation immediately in order to prevent clot propagation. If the block appears to resolve with this (i.e. pulses that were previously absent start to reappear), the collateral circulation may be producing an adequate distal blood supply. In this case, surgery may be avoided and the patient managed by thrombolysis (typically with tissue plasminogen activator alone). (For contraindications to thrombolysis, *see* p. 15.) However, if there is no improvement and the proximal pulses (popliteal, femoral or aortic) remain absent with neurological changes, surgery will be necessary. The vessel should be exposed and opened, and the clot removed using a Fogarty catheter. This is usually done in conjunction with an on-table arteriogram using femoral catheterisation. After successful embolectomy the precipitating cause (e.g. atrial fibrillation) should be dealt with.

Emboli in the upper limb vessels are usually less disabling (due to the fact that there is a better collateral circulation than in the lower limbs), and therefore less often require surgery. If there is no obvious cause of embolism, spontaneous thrombosis should be managed with thrombolysis plus angioplasty to deal with the underlying coronary disease.

If the acutely ischaemic limb is not managed promptly it will become gangrenous. The dead tissue appears black and wrinkled, and is painless, and the junction between dead and living tissue becomes well demarcated. If the dead tissue becomes infected, it will become soft and boggy with pus appearing at the line of demarcation (wet gangrene). Otherwise a hard, non-infected patch of dry gangrene results. This situation is irreversible, and the patient will require an amputation. It is important to remember that if amputation is deemed necessary it must be performed at a viable level. However, below-knee amputees recover function much better after rehabilitation than do through-knee or above-knee amputees.

Further reading

- Henke PK and Stanley JC (2004) The treatment of acute lower limb ischemia. *Adv Surg.* **38**: 281–91.
- Clagett GP, Sobel M, Jackson MR *et al.* (2004) Antithrombotic therapy in peripheral arterial occlusive disease: the Seventh American College of Chest Physicians Conference on Antithrombotic and Thrombolyic Therapy. *Chest.* **126 (Suppl. 3)**: 609–26S.
- Novo S, Coppola G and Milio G (2004) Critical limb ischemia: definition and natural history. *Curr Drug Targets Cardiovasc Haematol Disord.* **4**: 219–25.

10 Orthopaedics

Fractures

Fractures should be assessed after evaluating ABC (airway, breathing and circulation) in trauma patients. The commonest causes of fracture are road traffic accidents and falls, but repetitive stress (e.g. march fracture) and pathological causes (e.g. due to malignancy) also occur. In children, the fracture may not go from one cortex to the other (i.e. it may be incomplete). In major trauma, the fracture may be comminuted (with multiple bone fragments) or open (fracture site communicating with the overlying skin).

The main principles of fracture X-rays are as follows:

- always take two views of the whole bone, with the joint above and below the fracture
- if one bone of a pair is broken, look very carefully for a concomitant fracture of the other bone (e.g. radius and ulna, tibia and fibula)
- if there is no fracture, look for dislocation
- look for soft tissue injuries and foreign bodies.

The principles of fracture management are as follows:

- reduce (if necessary)
- hold (immobilise)
- rehabilitate.

A displaced fracture needs to be reduced back in place so that alignment of the fragments is achieved. This is especially important for fractures that go into joint lines (intra-articular fractures). If the fracture is not reduced with extreme precision, function will be impaired and the patient will suffer from secondary osteoarthritis. Once a fracture has been reduced satisfactorily, the reduction must be held in order to prevent slippage. Rehabilitation may involve exercises and physiotherapy. It is important to review patients regularly at the fracture clinic, and to assess the return of function as well as checking bone healing on X-ray.

Methods of reduction and immobilisation include traction, slings, splints and plaster casts, as well as operative approaches (internal and external fixation). The advantages of conservative methods are that they are relatively safe and simple, and there are no complications associated with surgery. However, it is more difficult to achieve and maintain a precise reduction, and the devices that are used can be quite cumbersome. Prolonged immobilisation can lead to pressure sores, thromboembolism and chest infection. Operative approaches, on the other hand, generally enable the patient to mobilise early and they allow a precise reduction that is held well.

In the emergency setting, an external fixation device may be applied quickly. A common example is the use of a ring external fixator to stabilise a pelvic fracture that has torn the internal iliac vessels and is causing serious haemodynamic compromise. As well as being simple, safe and fast, external fixation devices are associated with a lower risk of infection (although pin-track infection can occur) than internal fixation methods (e.g. plates, screws, intramedullary nails), and are therefore often used in open fractures. Internal fixation is usually more precise in reduction, and obviously is less cumbersome for the patient. However, the application of plates and screws, etc. requires an operation, and often the bone needs to be stripped of the surrounding soft tissue, which may compromise its blood supply. Infection of internal fixation devices is a serious complication and often necessitates removal of the metalwork.

Open fractures also require wound swabbing for culture, covering with povidone–iodine soaks, and photography (to avoid repeated examinations) before surgery to lavage and debride tissue as well as to reduce and hold the fracture. IV antibiotics (usually a third-generation cephalosporin with or without metronidazole if there is gross contamination) and tetanus prophylaxis (*see* p. 170) should be given.

Further reading

- Apley AG and Solomon L (2002) *Apley's System of Orthopaedics and Fractures* (8e). Butterworth-Heinemann, Oxford.
- McRae R (2001) *Pocketbook of Orthopaedics and Fractures*. Churchill Livingstone, Edinburgh.

Spinal injuries

Spinal cord injuries are commonly caused by shrapnel in military personnel, and by road traffic accidents, industrial or domestic accidents, and sports injuries in civilians. The thoracolumbar spine acts as a fulcrum and is therefore a common site of injury. Compression, distraction and shearing forces can all damage the spinal cord. A vertebral fracture may be stable (unlikely to damage the spinal cord) or unstable (spinal cord is already damaged, or likely to be damaged by subsequent movement). Whether the fracture is stable or not depends on the fracture pattern and the associated ligamentous injury.

Clinical features

There are many different types of cord injury:

- cord concussion (neuropraxia) – flaccid motor paralysis, sensory loss, and visceral paralysis below the level of injury; recovery is usually rapid and complete, starting within 8 hours
- cord transection – spinal shock (motor and visceral paralysis, sensory loss) is followed by reflex activity below the level of the lesion; the flaccid paralysis becomes spastic; recovery is minimal
- root transection – motor and visceral paralysis and sensory loss in the distribution of the damaged nerve roots; motor paralysis remains flaccid; recovery is variable
- cord syndromes:
  - central cord syndrome – hyperextension in elderly patients with pre-existing cervical osteoarthritis results in injury to the central grey matter with upper limb paralysis
  - anterior cord syndrome – damage to the anterior two-thirds of the cord leads to paralysis and loss of pain sensation, but spares the dorsal columns, so joint position sense and light touch are preserved
  - Brown–Sequard syndrome – hemisection of the cord causes ipsilateral paralysis and loss of joint position sense and light touch, and contralateral loss of pain sensation.

Cord injuries may be complete, with no function below the injured level, or incomplete, with some sparing of distal function. A full neurological assessment should be performed in patients who are at risk of cord injury. This includes assessment of anal tone, perianal sensation and abdominal reflexes.

Management

Evaluation of ABC (airway, breathing and circulation) according to Advanced Trauma Life Support (ATLS) guidelines is the priority. In 'A' the cervical spine should be controlled (*see* p. 149). The patient should be laid flat on a spinal board, and the vertebral column, anal tone and perianal sensation examined using a four-person log-roll technique. If there is damage to the spinal cord, closed reduction should be attempted immediately. For the cervical spine this is done with halo or tong traction, and for the thoracolumbar spine it is achieved with spinal bracing. Failing non-operative reduction, open reduction and segmental fixation using interspinous wires with single-level fusion are employed at specialist spinal units. Not only is surgery used to stabilise unstable fractures, but it is also indicated if there is cord compression with progression of symptoms (*see* p. 145). Autonomic disturbance (spinal shock) occurs as a result of damage to the sympathetic nervous system causing a decrease in sympathetic tone. This is manifested as peripheral vasodilatation, decreased blood pressure, decreased body temperature and, for lesions above T4 that supply the cardiac accelerator fibres, a decreased heart rate. Note how spinal shock differs from other shock states in that it involves bradycardia, making fluid resuscitation difficult. For this reason a urinary catheter and CVP line are usually necessary to tailor resuscitation. The use of high-dose methylprednisolone to limit spinal shock by reducing the oedema caused by the injury should be discussed with the neurosurgical team.

All patients with spinal cord injuries should be referred to specialist spinal units for further management and rehabilitation. This includes prevention of pressure sores (regular turning and getting the patient off the spinal board as soon as possible), chest physiotherapy and/or ventilatory support to prevent respiratory infections (for high lesions), limb physiotherapy to prevent joint contractures, bladder drainage, rectal disimpaction, and bladder retraining (bladder and bowel control is impaired in injuries above S2–4), as well as venous thromboprophylaxis, nutritional support and psychological counselling.

Further reading

- Kang AH (2005) Traumatic spinal cord injury. *Clin Obstet Gynecol.* **26**: 82–92.
- Sheerin F (2004) Spinal cord injury: anatomy and physiology of the spinal cord. *Emerg Nurs.* **12**: 30–6.
- Kirshblum S (2004) New rehabilitation interventions in spinal cord injury. *J Spinal Cord Med.* **27**: 342–50.

Cauda equina syndrome

The cauda equina is a 'horse's-tail'-like structure consisting of nerve roots exiting the end of the spinal cord to supply the lower limbs and pelvis. Compression of the nerve roots here results in lower limb weakness, bilateral sciatica (lumbar back pain that shoots down both legs), loss of perianal sensation and anal tone, and disturbance of bowel and bladder function (typically double incontinence, although urinary retention can also occur). The usual cause of this is a large, centrally prolapsed intervertebral disc (lower back pain, unilateral sciatica, and sensory disturbance without bowel or bladder dysfunction are commonly due to a laterally prolapsed intravertebral disc). However, it can also be due to spinal metastases (e.g. from lung, breast or prostate primaries), spinal cord tumours (e.g. myeloma, meningiomas and neurofibromas), vertebral bone disease (e.g. spondylolysis), syphilis and syringomyelia, although these more often cause a progressive compression of the spinal cord.

Signs of cauda equina syndrome should prompt immediate treatment with high-dose corticosteroids (e.g. 4 mg IV methylprednisolone), an urgent MRI scan to confirm the diagnosis, and then surgical decompression of the nerve roots. If these measures are not instituted within 6 hours, the patient is at high risk of permanent paralysis and incontinence. It is important that post-operatively the patient is taught isometric exercises and how to lie, sit, bend and lift with the least strain. This 'back schooling' will help to prevent chronic back pain, a common complication after back surgery.

Further reading

- Apley AG and Solomon L (2002) *Apley's System of Orthopaedics and Fractures* (8e). Butterworth-Heinemann, Oxford.
- McRae R (2001) *Pocketbook of Orthopaedics and Fractures*. Churchill Livingstone, Edinburgh.

Compartment syndrome

Compartment syndrome typically affects the forearm and lower limbs, but may also occasionally affect the abdomen and fingers. There are two anatomical compartments in the forearm, three in the thigh, and four in the leg, all composed of bones, interosseus membranes and investing layers of deep fascia. These compartments contain muscles, nerves and blood vessels.

Aetiology

A fracture can lead to bleeding, oedema or inflammation within one of these distinct compartments. Because the compartment has little room to expand, this will increase the intracompartmental pressure, reducing the capillary flow and causing muscle ischaemia. This itself worsens the oedema and leads to a vicious circle that culminates in nerve and muscle necrosis within 12 hours if the condition is left untreated. Nerves are capable of regeneration. However, infarcted muscle cannot regenerate, and instead it is replaced by inelastic fibrosis (Volkmann's ischaemic contracture).

Fractures are not the only cause of this limb-threatening cascade. Other causes include the following:

- crush injuries
- reperfusion injury
- prolonged limb compression (e.g. tight plaster cast, prolonged surgery)
- infection.

Clinical features

The clinical features of ischaemia are the six P's (*see* p. 139), but the diagnosis should be made before this stage. Ischaemic muscle is highly sensitive to stretch, so the patient who has a painful, swollen or tense muscle group with any of the above-mentioned causative factors should have these muscles stretched passively. If the pain is worsened, the diagnosis is confirmed. In doubtful cases, the intracompartmental pressure can be measured directly using a probe. If it is greater than 40 mmHg (with a normal diastolic blood pressure), the diagnosis is confirmed.

Management

The compartment must be decompressed immediately. Casts, bandages and dressings must be completely removed. If the intracompartmental pressure falls to below 40 mmHg, the limb may be closely monitored until the situation improves. If there is no improvement or the intracompartmental pressure does not fall to below 40 mmHg in the first place, then an open fasciotomy should be performed. In the leg (the commonest site of compartment syndrome), often all four compartments need to be decompressed. This can be done by removing a segment of fibula rather than decompressing each compartment in turn.

After decompression, the wound should be left open and inspected 5 days later. Any necrosed muscle can be debrided at this stage. Once the orthopaedic surgeon is satisfied that all of the remaining tissue is healthy, the wound can be closed in a tension-free manner (a skin graft may be required) or left to heal by secondary intention.

Further reading

- Apley AG and Solomon L (2002) *Apley's System of Orthopaedics and Fractures* (8e). Butterworth-Heinemann, Oxford.
- Kostler W, Strohm PC and Sudkamp NP (2004) Acute compartment syndrome of the limb. *Injury.* 35: 1221–7.

Acutely inflamed joint

The acutely painful, red, hot, swollen joint presents a diagnostic conundrum, including serious differential diagnoses. If more than one joint is affected, the cause is either viral or drug-induced polyarthropathy or a systemic disorder such as rheumatoid arthritis, Sjögren's syndrome, rheumatic fever, systemic lupus erythematosus, inflammatory bowel disease or psoriasis.

If only a single joint is inflamed, the potential causes include the above in addition to haemarthrosis (bleeding into the joint, usually as a result of trauma or haemophilia), gout, pseudogout and septic arthritis (i.e. infection). The patient will present with increased pain and inability to move the joint, general malaise and a spiking pyrexia, and the joint will exhibit the features of acute inflammation (dolor, calor, rubor and tumor). To make the diagnosis, it is vital to aspirate the joint (using aseptic technique to avoid introducing infection). Aspirated blood is likely to represent a haemarthrosis (or occasionally pseudogout). Fluid should be viewed under polarising light (in gout, negatively birefringent crystals are produced, whereas in pseudogout the crystals are positively birefringent). A haemarthrosis is usually managed conservatively with rest, analgesia, compression, elevation and ice packs. Acute gout and pseudogout are usually treated with NSAIDs.

The aspirated fluid (and pus) should also be sent for Gram staining and culture to look for evidence of septic arthritis, which can cause joint destruction and septicaemia, with potentially fatal consequences. The patient should therefore have bloods and blood cultures sent, and empirical IV antibiotics should be started immediately. In adults, usually flucloxacillin plus benzylpenicillin will cover the most likely causative organisms (S*taphylococcus*, *Streptococcus*, pneumococci and gonococci). In infants, *Haemophilus* is common, so a cephalosporin should also be given. In addition, the joint may benefit from a formal washout under general anaesthesia. The patient will also require strong analgesia and joint splinting in the position of optimum function (e.g. knee with 5–10 degrees of flexion to allow the foot to clear the ground when walking) for pain relief.

Further reading

- Apley AG and Solomon L (2002) *Apley's System of Orthopaedics and Fractures* (8e). Butterworth-Heinemann, Oxford.
- Smith CP and Hernon C (eds) (2000) *MRCS System Modules: essential revision notes.* Pastest, Knutsford.

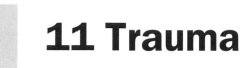

11 Trauma

Trauma: general principles

Trauma is the commonest cause of death in individuals aged 1–40 years in the UK. The distribution of trauma-related deaths is trimodal:

- 50% of deaths are 'immediate' (occurring within seconds or minutes), and are due to primary CNS injury or vascular lesions such as brainstem lacerations and aortic/large blood vessel lacerations
- 30% of deaths are 'early' (occurring within minutes or hours), and are due to uncontrolled blood loss or secondary CNS damage. It is in this 'early deaths' group that intervention can prevent mortality, for which reason this period is termed the 'golden hour'
- 20% of deaths are 'late' (occurring within days or weeks), and are caused by sepsis or multiple organ dysfunction syndrome (MODS) (see p. 255).

The Advanced Trauma Life Support (ATLS) system was developed in order to try to prevent morbidity and mortality in the 'golden hour'. It is divided into a primary survey, a secondary survey and a brief medical history. The trauma team usually consists of a general surgical registrar, an orthopaedic registrar and an A&E registrar, one or two A&E senior house officers, an anaesthetist, and two A&E nurses. Individuals who have completed the ATLS course are able to lead the team during a trauma call (this person is most often the A&E registrar).

Primary survey

The objective of the primary survey is to save life. Each of the following problems is dealt with in the order shown:

- *Airway:* check that the airway is patent and protect it. Ensure that the cervical spine is protected, especially in the unconscious or intoxicated patient with head or neck injuries.
- *Breathing:* check that there is adequate bilateral air entry and that there are no signs of life-threatening chest conditions (use the mnemonic

'ATOMFC': airway obstruction, tracheal disruption, open pneumothorax, massive haemothorax, flail chest and cardiac tamponade).

- *Circulation:* detect shock and treat it if present (*see* p. 156 and p. 250).
- *Disability:* examine the pupils for size, symmetry and response to
  light, and perform a brief neurological assessment using the 'AVPU'
  mnemonic:
  - A = alert
  - V = response to verbal stimuli
  - P = response to painful stimuli
  - U = unresponsive.
  Alternatively, a GCS examination can be performed at this stage (*see*
  p. 43).
- *Exposure:* completely undress the patient in order to inspect the
  entire body, including the spine.

Once the primary survey has been completed, some basic investigations
can be performed, such as blood glucose monitoring, baseline blood tests,
arterial blood gases, an electrocardiogram, and the trauma panel of
radiographs (chest, pelvis and/or lateral cervical spine). The trauma
team then progresses to the secondary survey.

Secondary survey

ABC (airway, breathing and circulation) is continually reassessed during
the secondary survey, and if there is any deterioration the primary survey
is started again from the beginning. The objective of the secondary survey
is to examine the patient thoroughly from head to toe, documenting
injuries as they are found, so that they can be dealt with at the end of the
survey. The secondary survey includes a digital rectal examination, a
vaginal examination in an adult female (with a female chaperone present), otorhinoscopy, and placement of a nasogastric tube (unless a skull
fracture is suspected) and a urinary catheter (unless a urethral injury is
suspected).

Medical history

If a medical history was not taken while performing the primary and
secondary surveys, it is appropriate to take an AMPLE history at this
point:

- Allergies.
- Medications.

- Past medical history.
- Last meal.
- Events leading to injury.

It is also important to check the patient's tetanus status and give prophylaxis if required (*see* p. 170).

Further reading

- American College of Surgeons (2003) *Advanced Trauma Life Support for Doctors: student course manual* (7e). American College of Surgeons, Chicago.

Trauma: airway

Inadequate delivery of oxygenated blood to the brain and heart is the quickest killer of the trauma patient. The prevention of hypoxia is therefore the first priority. The common causes of airway compromise are as follows:

- decreased GCS score (*see* p. 43) – head injury and drug or alcohol abuse are the usual precipitants
- maxillofacial trauma – trauma to the mid-face (classified as Le Fort injuries 1–3), as typically occurs after a road traffic accident in which an unbelted passenger or driver is thrown into the windscreen, can cause fracture-dislocations with disruption of the nasopharynx and oropharynx. This, together with associated bleeding, increased secretions and dislodged teeth, makes airway compromise likely
- neck injuries – penetrating injuries can damage vessels and cause displacement and obstruction of the airway. Direct damage to the larynx or trachea can also occur
- laryngeal trauma – hoarseness, subcutaneous (surgical) emphysema and a palpable fracture are signs of laryngeal fracture.

It is vital to be able to recognise a compromised airway. A patient who is able to talk without difficulty is likely to have a secure airway.

- **Look** for facial/airway trauma, agitation, cyanosis and the use of accessory muscles of ventilation.
- **Listen** for stridor, gurgling noises, snoring or hoarseness.
- **Feel** for chest wall movement with breathing.

Administer supplemental oxygen at a rate of 15 litres/minute with a reservoir (re-breathe) bag. Do not worry about carbon dioxide retention in chronic obstructive airways disease – hypoxia kills much more quickly than hypercapnoea in the trauma patient.

If the airway is obstructed, clear any physical obstruction (teeth, foreign body or tongue), and then maintain the airway in an unobstructed position using the chin-lift and jaw-thrusts manoeuvres, and by inserting an oropharyngeal (Guedel) airway (a nasopharyngeal airway is an alternative, except in cases of facial trauma, where brain injury may result from its use). It is important to reassess the airway after these initial attempts at securing it. If it is still inadequate, a definitive airway is needed. Definitive airways include orotracheal (conventional) intubation, nasotracheal intubation and surgical airways (cricothyroidotomy and tracheostomy), which should be performed by skilled anaesthetists in the trauma patient.

After the airway has been secured, it is vital to secure the cervical spinal cord. Any trauma patient with an injury above the clavicle should be assumed to have a cervical spine injury. This is stabilised by the use of in-line immobilisation and a 'CSF' – a collar (different-sized neck collars are available), sandbags (to support the head on either side) and forehead taping (to secure the sandbags and collar to the spinal board). If the cervical spine is not protected, any movement may cause injury to the underlying spinal cord, with resulting paralysis. It is important to remember that although lateral cervical spine X-rays may show disruption of the normal alignment of the neck, cervical spine injury may be present with a normal X-ray. Therefore the cervical spine should always be immobilised if the mechanism of injury is suspicious. During the secondary survey, if there is no sign of cervical spine injury on examination, the 'CSF' can be removed.

Once the airway and cervical spine have been secured and the other priorities (breathing, circulation, the secondary survey, etc.) dealt with, any fracture or disruption can be managed by specialists in order to restore the integrity of the damaged airway.

Further reading

- American College of Surgeons (2003) *Advanced Trauma Life Support for Doctors: student course manual* (7e). American College of Surgeons, Chicago.

Trauma: breathing

If ventilation is not adequate after the airway has been secured, ventilatory support may be needed. This can be assessed by pulse oximetry to measure oxygen saturations, which should be above 92% in order to maintain an adequate partial pressure of oxygen in the blood. This is seen from the sigmoid-shaped oxyhaemoglobin dissociation curve. With a secure airway, ventilation (breathing) may still be compromised by direct chest trauma, intracranial injury or cervical spinal cord injury. Ventilatory support may be delivered via mouth-to-mouth, mouth-to-mask, bag-and-mask or intermittent positive pressure ventilation after endotracheal intubation (this may require paralysis and sedation of the patient by an anaesthetist).

Signs of inadequate ventilation include apnoea (due to neuromuscular paralysis or being unconscious), tachypnoea, decreased oxygen saturations, hypoxia or hypercarbia on ABG monitoring, and cyanosis. If the chest does not rise and fall symmetrically, this suggests splinting or a flail chest. Decreased or absent breath sounds over one or both hemithoraces suggest that a thoracic injury is present.

Thoracic injuries

The following thoracic injuries should be recognised and managed in the primary survey.

- *Tension pneumothorax.* This develops when a 'one-way-valve' air leak occurs from the lung or chest wall, causing collapse of the affected lung, and subsequent mediastinal shift to the opposite side. The patient will show signs of ventilatory compromise, absent breath sounds on the side of the tension pneumothorax, and a tracheal (mediastinal) shift to the opposite side. These signs indicate an urgent need for decompression with a large-bore needle (e.g. a grey venflon) into the second intercostal space in the mid-clavicular line of the affected hemithorax. There is no time to confirm the diagnosis with an X-ray. Following the sound of a hiss indicating successful decompression (the sound of a life saved!), a chest drain should be inserted into the fifth intercostal space (at nipple level) between the anterior and mid-axillary lines.
- *Open pneumothorax.* Large chest wall defects can cause a sucking chest wound in which air passes through the chest defect with each breath rather than down the trachea, leading to inadequate ventilation. The defect should be closed with a sterile occlusive dressing taped

down on three sides to produce a flutter valve. When the patient breathes in, the dressing is sucked over the wound, thereby preventing air from entering. On exhalation, the open end of the dressing allows air to escape. After this, a definitive chest drain should be inserted and the defect closed surgically.

- *Flail chest*. Here there is a segment of the chest wall that is not in continuity with the rest of the bony thorax. This can occur after multiple rib fractures in multiple sites on the same ribs. The flail segment will move in the opposite direction to the rest of the bony thorax during breathing, which results in poor ventilation. The underlying lung may also be contused, which worsens the problem. The diagnosis can be made by observing the paradoxical movement of the flail chest, by palpating crepitus of rib fractures, or by observing the fractures on a chest X-ray. ABG monitoring will indicate hypoxia. Supportive measures such as analgesia, oxygenation, fluid resuscitation and/or the use of a ventilator may be required.
- *Massive haemothorax*. The filling of the chest with more than 1.5 litres of blood will compress the lungs and prevent adequate breathing. A chest drain is required. The patient may also exhibit signs of circulatory compromise (*see* p. 250).

Further reading

- American College of Surgeons (2003) *Advanced Trauma Life Support for Doctors: student course manual* (7e). American College of Surgeons, Chicago.

Trauma: circulation

Haemorrhage is one of the commonest causes of shock, and leads to a loss of circulating blood and fluid (hypovolaemic shock). It should always be suspected in any case of haemodynamic compromise due to major trauma. Severe haemorrhage may not always be easy to recognise. Possible locations of such 'hidden haemorrhage' include the thorax, the abdomen (especially the retroperitoneal space), pelvic fractures, or blood spilt at the site of injury (i.e. 'in the chest, in the belly, or on the road').

Management

After stabilisation of 'A' (airway) and 'B' (breathing), 'C' (circulation) is managed by controlling any obvious sources of bleeding with direct pressure and elevation, fluid replacement and cardiac support. Fluid can be replaced intravenously after the insertion of two large-bore (grey/brown) cannulae into large peripheral (e.g. antecubital fossa) veins. If initial access is difficult, a cutdown on to the great saphenous vein can be performed, although in children under 8 years of age it is often quicker to insert an intraosseus cannula into the femur or tibia. Once access has been obtained, fluid should be given as quickly as possible initially, and then titrated to the patient's clinical response.

The question of what replacement fluid to use is a matter of debate. Crystalloids are fluids that do not contain proteins, and colloids are fluids that do. Colloids are therefore more 'physiological' (i.e. more like the plasma that the patient has lost) and thus in theory might seem more attractive to use. However, they do not remain in the circulation as long as crystalloids, and they may uncommonly cause an anaphylactoid reaction. Fluid resuscitation could begin with colloid, in order to increase the circulating volume rapidly, and then move on to crystalloids to maintain it. Typically, in resuscitation, gelofusine is the colloid of choice (although occasionally haemaccel is used), and the crystalloid of choice is normal (isotonic) saline (0.9%) or Hartmann's solution (also known as Ringer's lactate). However, volume of fluid is more important than the specific fluid used.

In severe haemorrhage, blood transfusion may be needed, and therefore at the time of IV cannulation it is important to send blood for cross-matching (as well as for assay of haemoglobin, glucose, renal function, etc.). It takes about 1 hour to prepare fully cross-matched blood. In an emergency, type-specific blood (which takes 10 minutes to prepare) or type O blood (universal donor, as it has no antigens and can be given to anyone) is used instead. It is important to remember that if not fully cross-matched, rhesus-negative blood must be used in female patients of childbearing age.

Whatever type of fluid resuscitation is employed, the fluid should be warmed towards body temperature before infusion in order to avoid making the patient hypothermic.

A surgical opinion should be sought early in the resuscitation process in order to try to identify the cause of bleeding, and to decide whether further investigations (e.g. CT scanning) or surgical intervention (e.g. laparotomy) are required. The value of diagnostic peritoneal lavage is controversial in units with rapid access to a CT scanner.

(For information on cardiac support and response monitoring, *see* pp. 251–2.)

Further reading

- Shafi S and Kauder DR (2004) Fluid resuscitation and blood replacement in patients with polytrauma. *Clin Orthop.* **422**: 37–42.
- Archbold A (2001) Management of haemorrhage and shock In: R Ashford and N Evans (eds) *Surgical Critical Care.* Greenwich Medical Media Ltd, London.

Head injury

Each year over a million patients present to Accident and Emergency departments in the UK with head injuries. Assaults and road traffic accidents are the major causes of such injury, with alcohol or other drugs being a frequent co-factor.

Glasgow Coma Scale (GCS)

This universally used scoring system is used to assess consciousness (*see* p. 43).

A GCS score of ≤ 8 is the definition of coma and is an indication for obtaining a definitive airway (e.g. with an endotracheal tube). A mild head injury is one associated with a GCS score of 13–15, a moderate head injury has a GCS score of 9–12, and a severe head injury has a GCS score of ≤ 8.

Pathophysiology

Primary brain injury occurs on impact, due to shearing forces that cause tearing of axonal tracts. There is little that can be done to minimise the consequences of primary brain injury, and management is therefore aimed at preventing secondary effects.

Secondary brain injury may follow primary brain injury because of the following:

- extracranial causes – hypoxia due to airway obstruction, loss of respiratory drive or pulmonary complications (e.g. acute respiratory distress syndrome), and hypotension resulting from shock due to coexisting injuries
- intracranial causes – due to raised intracranial pressure (ICP). The addition of a space-occupying lesion (e.g. extradural haematoma, cerebral oedema) within the constant intracranial volume will eventually result in an exponential increase in ICP once the brain's autoregulatory mechanisms are saturated. This will result in a decrease in cerebral perfusion pressure, causing the blood flow to the brain to become compromised, with subsequent ischaemic damage. The raised ICP compresses the oculomotor nerve (cranial nerve III), causing pupillary dilatation, and compresses the corticospinal tracts, causing motor weakness. The pressure eventually compresses the brainstem (a process known as 'coning') and the vital cardio-respiratory centre, resulting in death.

Management

ABC is the priority, and once it is stabilised 'D' (neurological disability) is assessed using the GCS. The trend in the GCS score, indicating deterioration, stability or improvement, is often more important than the absolute value, and for this reason the GCS should be assessed regularly. CT or MRI imaging can then be performed based on the scores obtained. A skull X-ray is not indicated in the management of head injury, based on current guidelines.

Indications for a CT scan

- Loss of consciousness or a deteriorating GCS score.
- A period of amnesia.
- Neurological symptoms and/or signs.
- CSF otorrhoea or rhinorrhoea (CSF flowing from the ears or nose).
- Severe scalp injury or clinical suspicion of fracture.
- Suspected penetrating injury.
- Pupillary signs.
- Focal neurological signs.
- The conscious level does not improve with time.
- The conscious level is difficult to assess (e.g. the patient is intoxicated).

Indications for hospital admission

- Loss of consciousness for longer than 5 minutes (or amnesia).
- GCS score of < 13 or decreasing GCS score.
- Skull fracture.
- Neurological symptoms and/or signs.
- Worsening headache, nausea or vomiting.
- Extensive laceration.
- The conscious level is difficult to assess (e.g. due to alcohol intoxication).
- No responsible carer at home.
- Other medical conditions (e.g. clotting abnormalities).

A neurosurgical opinion should be sought early if there is any suspicion of an intracranial injury. Early endotracheal intubation should be performed on all patients with a severe head injury (GCS score ≤ 8), as it has been shown to reduce the development of secondary brain injury.

Specific management strategies to control intracranial pressure, maintain cerebral perfusion pressure and reduce the cerebral metabolic rate for oxygen can be instituted after neurosurgical consultation, but only in an ITU setting with ICP-monitoring facilities.

Further reading

- Ledingham IMA (ed.) (2000) Altered consciousness/confusion (Critical Care – Module 1). In: *RCSE SELECT Programme.* Centre for Medical Education, University of Dundee, Dundee.
- Kirk R, Mansfield A and Cochrane P (eds) (1999) *Clinical Surgery in General* (3e). Churchill Livingstone, London.
- Downs R (2001) Head injury. In: R Ashford and N Evans (eds) *Surgical Critical Care.* Greenwich Medical Media Ltd, London.

Drowning and hypothermia

Drowning

Drowning and near drowning are important causes of death worldwide. There are an estimated half a million episodes each year, the majority of which are preventable.

- Drowning may be defined as death caused by suffocation by sub mersion in a liquid.
- Near drowning is survival (even if only temporary) from suffocation by submersion in a liquid.

Aetiology

- In the majority of cases fluid is aspirated into the lungs.
- This causes pulmonary vasoconstriction and a rapid decline in cardiac output, leading to secondary cardiac arrest.
- If submersion occurs in icy water (< 5°C), there is rapid cooling with the onset of hypothermia. This may give a degree of protection from anoxia (mainly in children).
- Following near drowning there is a high risk of respiratory complications such as acute respiratory distress syndrome.

Management

- When rescuing drowning victims, attention must also be focused on the safety of the rescuers.
- Consider the risk of spinal injuries.
- Resuscitation should begin at the scene.
- Clear the airway. In unconscious patients, intubate early (as there is a high risk of vomiting).
- Give all patients supplemental oxygen. Many patients will require further respiratory support.
- A nasogastric tube should be sited to empty the stomach.
- Patients may suffer circulatory collapse after rescue (the liquid exerts a hydrostatic pressure on the body which is removed at the time of rescue). Intravenous fluids may need to be administered.
- Start rewarming the patient (*see* below).
- Investigations should include fluid and electrolyte balance, blood gases, ECG and chest X-ray.

- If cardiac arrest occurs, commence cardiopulmonary resuscitation and follow the appropriate arrest protocol. Most patients are also hypothermic, and the principles described below should be observed.
- Asymptomatic patients should be monitored for at least 6 hours before discharge, as there is a 10% risk of late deterioration.

Prognosis

- Up to 25% of patients who present to the Accident and Emergency department will die, and 6% will suffer neurological deficits.
- Patients who are in sinus rhythm, have reactive pupils and show good neurological responsiveness at the scene have better survival outcomes.

Hypothermia

- Hypothermia is diagnosed when the core body temperature falls below 35°C. It may be classified as shown in Table 22.

Table 22   Classification of hypothermia

Severity	Temperature (°C)
Mild	32–35
Moderate	30–32
Severe	< 30

- A low-reading thermometer is required. Tympanic and oesophageal probes best reflect the true core temperature. Rectal thermometers may also be used.

Risk factors

- Environmental insult (e.g. immersion in cold water, hill walking in wet and windy conditions).
- Infants.
- The elderly.
- Excess alcohol ingestion.
- Hypothyroidism.
- Immobility.
- Malnutrition.
- Infections.

Clinical features

Table 23 Clinical features of hypothermia

Mild	Moderate	Severe
Shivering	Muscular rigidity	Cardiac arrest
Aggression	Hypotension	Ventricular fibrillation
Confusion	Arrhythmias	may occur spontaneously
Drowsiness	Decreased level of	below 28°C
Ataxia	consciousness	
Dysarthria	Coma	

Investigations

- FBC.
- Clotting (hypothermia may cause clotting disturbance).
- U&Es (hyperkalaemia may occur during rewarming).
- Glucose (hypoglycaemia may be a precipitating cause).
- Thyroid function tests.
- Amylase (pancreatitis is a recognised complication).
- Blood cultures.
- Blood gases.
- Chest X-ray (look for evidence of pneumonia or heart failure).
- ECG (bradycardia and atrial fibrillation are the commonest arrhythmias and may precede ventricular fibrillation).
- CT scan of the head (may be indicated if there is a possibility of head injury or stroke).

Management

- Remove the individual from the cold environment.
- Assess ABC.
- Give warmed, humidified oxygen.
- Obtain intravenous access.
- Consider a slow intravenous infusion. The patient may show evidence of hypovolaemia as rewarming occurs (because the vascular spaces will expand due to vasodilation). However, caution is required, as patients (especially the elderly) are also at risk of pulmonary oedema.
- Perform continuous cardiac monitoring.
- Correct any underlying causes (e.g. give antibiotics to treat infections).

Rewarming

- Mild cases may be rewarmed passively by wrapping the patient in warm blankets in a warm room.
- More severe cases will require the following active measures:
  - external – warm baths, wrapping in a hot air blanket
  - internal – including gastric, bladder, thoracic and peritoneal lavage with warmed fluids. Cardiopulmonary bypass, if available, is the method of choice for patients with severe hypothermia or those who have suffered a cardiac arrest.
- The rate of rewarming should be approximately 1–2°C per hour. However, it should be slower in the elderly (0.5°C per hour), as they are at increased risk of cerebral and pulmonary oedema with rapid rewarming.

Cardiac arrest

- Hypothermia protects the brain and organs, so prolonged resuscitative attempts are indicated.
- Cardiopulmonary resuscitation should be performed with a ratio of 30 compressions to 2 ventilations.
- The patient should be rewarmed rapidly; cardiopulmonary bypass may achieve rewarming of 1–2°C every 5 minutes.
- Consider a single shock if the patient is in ventricular fibrillation, but if they are unresponsive no further shocks should be administered until the core temperature is at least 30°C.
- Drugs are also usually withheld until the core temperature is at least 30°C (there is often no response at lower temperatures, and the drugs may accumulate to toxic levels during rewarming).
- Death may be difficult to diagnose. *Remember that the patient is not dead until they are warm and dead.* Resuscitation should be continued until the core temperature is at least 32°C (or until it cannot be raised despite active measures).

Further reading

- Resuscitation Council (UK) (2005) *Adult Basic Life Support*. Resuscitation Council (UK), London; www.resus.org.uk/pages/bls.pdf
- Resuscitation Council (UK) and European Resuscitation Council (2004) *Advanced Life Support Manual* (4e revised). Resuscitation Council (UK) and European Resuscitation Council, London.
- Warrell D, Cox TM, Firth JD *et al.* (2003) *Oxford Textbook of Medicine* (4e). Oxford University Press, Oxford.

12 Plastic surgery/ dermatology

Burns

Clinical features

Burns can be classified by type (thermal, electrical or chemical) or by depth (partial or full thickness). An electrical burn is always full thickness and is usually far more extensive than its external appearance would suggest. A partial-thickness burn does not penetrate through the underlying germinal layer and is therefore more superficial than a full-thickness burn. Because of this, partial-thickness burns have an intact sensation and are thus painful, unlike many full-thickness burns in which the nerve endings are destroyed. Partial-thickness burns heal completely within a few days, whereas full-thickness burns scar and contract. Partial-thickness burns also blister, in contrast to full-thickness burns, in which slough on top of granulation tissue predominates. Loss of the epidermis in burns means that there is exudation of plasma, so electrolyte imbalance and shock may occur.

Respiratory obstruction can result from smoke inhalation or thermal injury to the airways. Signs of this include singeing of nasal hair, soot around the nose and mouth, coughing, and signs of respiratory distress (e.g. increased respiratory rate, use of accessory muscles). The stress response of the body can lead to sodium and water retention, potassium loss and protein catabolism, as well as peptic ulceration (Curling's ulcers). The release of toxins from the burn can result in toxaemia, but this is rare if the burn is managed adequately.

Management

First, evaluate ABC. If the airway is compromised by laryngeal oedema from a respiratory burn, early endotracheal intubation should be considered, and an anaesthetist should be informed immediately. Carboxyhaemoglobin levels should be checked if carbon monoxide poisoning is suspected (this is managed supportively with high-flow oxygen and occasionally the use of hyperbaric oxygenation and ventilatory support). The burn should be cooled by applying cold running water to it, and the wound should be cleaned and dressed with silver sulphadiazine cream to prevent infection, and covered with clingfilm to minimise plasma loss and prevent air from flowing over the burn, thus providing some pain relief. Analgesia should be given (IV opiates are often required).

Full-thickness burns are best treated by immediate excision of the burned area (escharectomy) and split-skin grafting, which help to prevent infection. If the full-thickness burn is circumferential, this can lead to compartment syndrome (*see* p. 146), or it may restrict breathing if the chest is compressed. In these situations incision of the eschar (escharotomy) becomes urgent, and this can be followed by a full escharectomy later.

If the surface area of the burn is extensive, the plastic surgeon may have to use donor skin from a relative or human skin bank (allograft), or temporarily skin from a pig (xenograft), for the skin graft. More recently, skin from tissue culture has been used. Skin grafting is performed immediately for the eyelids in order to avoid ectropion and corneal ulceration. Next in priority are the face, hands and joint creases, as scarring at these sites will cause significant disability and deformity.

Because of the catabolic stress response to the burn, the patient may require increased nutritional intake to avoid going into a negative nitrogen balance. This should be commenced within 24 hours of the burn. If the gastrointestinal tract is unaffected, enteral nutrition is always preferred, otherwise parenteral nutrition should be used.

The management of shock and fluid balance in patients with burns can be complex. It is important to work out the amount of fluid replacement required and to use the correct type of replacement fluid. The severely burned patient will lose plasma most rapidly within the first 12 hours, and therefore replacement should start as soon as possible. Obviously the larger the area of epidermis that is lost, the greater the amount of fluid that will be lost and which will therefore need to be replaced. The 'rule of nines' is used to estimate the area of the burn (*see* Figure 14 opposite).

This rule is useful for adults, but it is not so accurate in children and infants, whose heads have a proportionately larger surface area. Special charts for estimating the burned surface area in these cases are available. Burns exceeding 10% of body surface area in children and 15% of that in adults usually require IV fluid replacement (smaller burns can be

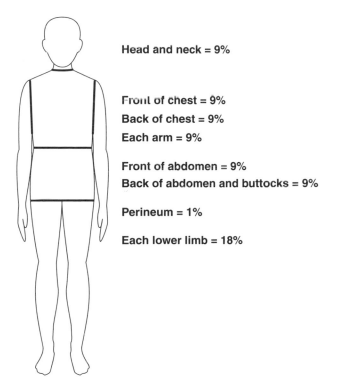

Head and neck = 9%

Front of chest = 9%
Back of chest = 9%
Each arm = 9%

Front of abdomen = 9%
Back of abdomen and buttocks = 9%

Perineum = 1%

Each lower limb = 18%

Figure 14 The rule of nines

managed with oral intake). Many protocols exist, but the Mount Vernon formula is a simple guide that is easy to remember:

$$\text{Fluid replacement (ml) per period} = \frac{\text{weight (kg) x burn area (\%)}}{2}.$$

This calculated volume of fluid is given every 4 hours for the first 12 hours, every 6 hours for the next 12 hours, and then 12-hourly for the next 12 hours. This is in addition to the patient's normal maintenance fluid requirement of 3 litres of crystalloid for an adult. As the fluid that is lost is plasma, it should be replaced with colloid (e.g. Hartmann's solution). Roughly half the fluid volume should be replaced with a blood transfusion if the burn is full thickness, as there will be extensive red blood cell destruction in these cases. It should be noted that the Mount Vernon formula and the 'rule of nines' are merely guides, and fluid resuscitation should be tailored to the urinary output, heart rate, blood pressure and CVP as appropriate (*see* p. 251).

Burns to the airway, significant full-thickness burns, burns exceeding 10% of the surface area in children or 15% of that in adults, and burns to the eyes, face, hands and perineum should all be referred to a specialist burns unit for further management. This reduces the mortality and morbidity in these cases, which have a poor prognosis.

Further reading

- Ellis H, Calne R and Watson C (1998) *Lecture Notes in General Surgery* (9e). Blackwell Science, Oxford.
- Demling RH and Seigne P (2000) Metabolic management of patients with severe burns. *World J Surg.* **24**: 673–80.
- Yowler CJ and Fratianne RB (2000) Current status of burn resuscitation. *Clin Plast Surg.* **27**: 1–10.

Wounds

Wounds may have medico-legal implications, so clinical notes should be legible, thorough and accurate. Wounds can be caused by trauma or surgery. After management of ABC and the application of direct pressure to the wound to stop bleeding, the wound should be assessed in terms of its site, length and associated injuries (e.g. fractures, nerve, tendon or vascular injuries). It should be swabbed for culture if there are signs of inflammation (*see* p. 254). Adequate analgesia should be given to the patient before the wound is explored. The maximum safe dose of lidocaine is 1 mg/kg (or 3 mg/kg if used with epinephrine). When applying local anaesthetic it is important to withdraw the syringe plunger before the lidocaine is applied, to ensure that the injection is not intravascular. Local anaesthesia is often not appropriate for children who cannot remain still and calm, and who therefore often require general anaesthetic for exploration. Wound exploration must be performed in a sterile manner and any foreign bodies should be removed. Any neurovascular or tendon injury, or foreign body that cannot be removed, should prompt referral to a specialist for operative management.

If a fracture is suspected, X-rays should be taken. If the fracture is confirmed then it is termed 'open'. These wounds always require thorough lavage and debridement, and should be referred to an orthopaedic surgeon rather than closed primarily in Accident and Emergency (*see* p. 142). Irrigation with normal saline is usually appropriate, and pressure irrigation by squeezing the bag will help to remove any dirt. Primary closure should only be considered for wounds that have no associated injuries and a low risk of infection. As the risk of infection rises with increasing duration of exposure of the wound to the exterior, primary closure is not usually performed for wounds that are more than 6 hours old. Delayed primary closure after 3–5 days, or no intervention at all (allowing the wound to heal by secondary intention), should be considered in this situation.

Wounds can be classified on the basis of the risk of infection. Clean wounds are incisions through non-inflamed tissue with no entry into the respiratory, gastrointestinal or genito-urinary tracts. They include simple lacerations, and the risk of infection is less than 2%. Clean–contaminated wounds are those in which there is entry into a hollow viscus other than the large bowel, with minimal contamination. These have a risk of sepsis of 2–10%. In contaminated wounds the hollow viscus is breached, with more spillage (e.g. operations that open the colon, open fractures and dog bites), and the risk of infection is 10–30%. Dirty wounds are associated with pus, a perforated viscus (e.g. faecal peritonitis) or traumatic wounds more than 6 hours old, and the risk of sepsis is over 30%.

Contaminated and dirty wounds require antibiotic prophylaxis to prevent infection. The choice of regime is tailored according to the bacteria that are most likely to need targeting, and individual protocols vary from one hospital to another. In skin breaches, oral flucloxacillin plus penicillin V is usually appropriate to prevent staphyloccocal and streptococcal infection. In colonic surgery, antibiotics that cover anaerobes (e.g. metronidazole) are required. If the wound is planned (i.e. surgical), it is important to ensure that antibiotic prophylaxis is started early enough to ensure that there are adequate drug levels in the circulation at the time of surgical incision. This usually means that antibiotics must be started before or at the time of anaesthetic induction.

In addition to antibiotic prophylaxis, thorough lavage together with debridement of devitalised tissue, the removal of foreign bodies, attention to sterility and the avoidance of early primary closure, it is important to consider tetanus prophylaxis. Contaminated and dirty wounds, those with devitalised tissue or signs of infection, wounds that are over 6 hours old, and puncture wounds are all 'tetanus prone'. These require a tetanus toxoid booster if the patient has had a booster within the last 10 years, or a booster plus human anti-tetanus immunoglobulin (HATI) if the patient has not had a booster for more than 10 years. If the patient with a 'tetanus-prone' wound has never had the tetanus immunisation as a baby, it is reasonable to start the course (to be completed with their GP) and to give HATI as well. No prophylaxis against tetanus is needed in patients with clean wounds who have had a booster within the last 10 years. Those who have not had a booster for more than 10 years should be given another one, and those who never received the initial tetanus course should be given their first injection of the course, and then complete the course with their GP.

Further reading

- Elkabir JJ and Khadra A (1999) *MRCS Core Modules: essential revision notes.* Pastest, Knutsford.
- Sooriakumaran P, Jayasena C and Scully C (2005) *Key Topics in Human Diseases for Dental Students.* Taylor & Francis, London.

Erythroderma

Clinical features

Erythroderma may be defined as any inflammatory skin disease that affects more than 90% of the body surface. Patchy erythema generalises rapidly and may be accompanied by systemic upset, including fever, shivering and malaise. The skin is bright red, hot, dry and thickened. Patients may complain of itching or more frequently 'tightness' of the skin. Scaling appears after 2–6 days, and varying degrees of lymphadenopathy are present.

Aetiology

- Eczema – more common in the elderly, but can occur at any age in atopic individuals.
- Psoriasis – may be precipitated by treatment with potent topical or systemic steroids.
- Drugs – many drugs can cause erythroderma. The commonest culprits are gold, cimetidine, carbamazepine, lithium, and occasionally penicillin and barbiturates.
- Lymphoma and leukaemias – cutaneous T-cell lymphoma is seen most often, followed by Hodgkin's disease. Cases have been reported with non-Hodgkin's lymphoma, leukaemia and myelodysplasia.
- Rarer causes include the following:
  - pemphigus
  - dermatomyositis
  - lichen planus
  - pemphigoid
  - sarcoidosis.

Complications

- Thermoregulation – control may be lost, with patients becoming hypothermic due to increased skin perfusion.
- High-output cardiac failure – especially in elderly patients, due to increased blood flow through the skin.
- Dehydration – due to increased fluid loss by transpiration.
- Hypoalbuminaemia – decreased synthesis and increased metabolism of albumin, and increased protein loss via scaling of the skin.
- Electrolyte disturbances.

- Infections – cutaneous and respiratory infections are common, and are a frequent cause of mortality.

Management

- Identify the cause, via history, skin biopsy and lymph node biopsy (if lymphoma is suspected).
- Admit the patient to hospital, as there is a risk of complications.
- Regulate the environmental temperature (cooling and overheating should be avoided by using blankets or fans).
- Monitor the fluid and electrolyte balance and maintain adequate fluid intake.
- Treat cardiac failure if it develops.
- Consider drug reaction as a possible cause, and withdraw all non-essential drugs.
- Treat the skin with emollients.
- Mild topical steroids may be used, but there is a risk of exacerbating psoriatic erythroderma with potent or systemic steroids.

Prognosis

- Erythroderma is a serious disease, and death rates of 18–64% have been reported. Cutaneous and respiratory infections are common. Mortality is highest in the elderly.
- Erythroderma caused by drugs has the best prognosis, with many cases resolving within 2–6 weeks after the drug has been withdrawn.
- Other forms may continue for months to years, and relapse is common.
- T-cell lymphoma may develop years after initial presentation with erythroderma.

Further reading

- Champion RH, Burton JL, Burns BA and Breathnach SM (eds) (1998) *Textbook of Dermatology* (6e). Blackwell Science, Oxford.

Stevens–Johnson's syndrome

Classification

There has been much debate about the exact classification of Stevens–Johnson's syndrome. In 1922, Stevens and Johnson described a new syndrome consisting of fever, erosive stomatitis, severe purulent conjunctivitis and a disseminated cutaneous eruption. They believed this to be a new disease entity. However, Stevens–Johnson's syndrome later became synonymous with erythema multiforme major (skin lesions with the involvement of two mucous membranes).

It has been suggested that erythema multiforme major and Stevens–Johnson's syndrome represent two distinct syndromes (*see* Table 24).

Table 24   Signs and symptoms of erythema multiforme major and Stevens–Johnson's syndrome

Erythema multiforme major	*Stevens–Johnson's syndrome*
Classic target lesions	Atypical target lesions
Acral distribution	Non-acral distribution
Inflammatory dermal histology	Epidermal necrolysis predominates
Association with viral infections	Association with drug sensitivity

In the past decade there has been an increasing tendency to classify Stevens–Johnson's syndrome along the same disease spectrum as toxic epidermal necrolysis (TENS). It has been proposed that the two conditions be distinguished on the basis of the extent of cutaneous involvement. In TENS there is epidermal loss over more than 30% of the body surface, in Stevens–Johnson's syndrome there is less than 10% loss, and cases in between are classified as TEN-Stevens–Johnson's syndrome overlap.

Aetiology

- The majority of cases are caused by drugs, including sulphonamides, anticonvulsants, non-steroidal anti-inflammatory drugs, allopurinol, tetracyclines and penicillins. The exact mechanism involved is unknown, but it is believed that it is likely to be a hypersensitivity reaction.

- Stevens–Johnson's syndrome is occasionally related to infections (herpes viruses and *Mycoplasma pneumoniae*).

Clinical features

- Fever.
- Malaise.
- Myalgia.
- Arthralgia.
- Skin lesions – maculopapular lesions, bullae and erosions covering less than 10% of the body's surface area.
- Mucosal involvement:
  - characteristic haemorrhagic crusting of the lips and mouth
  - severe conjunctivitis
  - corneal ulceration
  - genital lesions.

Complications

- Skin failure:
  - loss of temperature control
  - fluid and electrolyte imbalance
  - failure of mechanical barrier.
- Secondary infection.
- Respiratory symptoms.
- Renal involvement.

Management

- There is no specific treatment available, and management is supportive.
- Any drugs suspected of precipitating the condition should be withdrawn.
- Good nursing care is of paramount importance, and patients may need to be cared for on dermatological intensive-care or burns units.
- Electrolyte and fluid balance should be monitored and maintained.
- Nutritional support via a nasogastric tube may be required until the oral mucosa has healed.
- Ophthalmological review is important to minimise the (rare) risk of permanent eye damage and blindness.
- Topical emollients should be used to soothe the skin.
- Analgesia should be given (opiates are often required).

- Antibiotics may be necessary to treat secondary infection.
- The use of steroids remains controversial. Although it is considered that they may be of some benefit during the initial phase of the disease, there have been reports of increased morbidity and mortality due to an increased risk of sepsis.
- Case reports suggest that intravenous immunoglobulin may be a useful therapy, but clinical trials are required.

Prognosis

Mortality rates of approximately 5% have been reported. Infection is the main cause of death.

Further reading

- Champion RH, Burton JL, Burns BA and Breathnach SM (eds) (1998) *Textbook of Dermatology* (6e). Blackwell Science, Oxford.
- Craven NM (2000) Management of toxic epidermal necrolysis. *Hosp Med.* **61:** 778–81.
- Merry DW, Jung P and Levy ML (2003) Use of intravenous immunoglobulin in children with Stevens–Johnson syndrome and toxic epidermal necrolysis: seven cases and review of the literature. *Pediatrics.* **112:** 1430–6.

13 Ophthalmology/ otorhinolaryngology

Red eye

Differential diagnosis

- Haemorrhage.
- Conjunctivitis.
- Corneal disease.
- Iridocyclitis.
- Acute glaucoma.
- Optic neuritis.

Practical approach

- Determine whether red eye is due to haemorrhage or congestion (vasodilation of vessels).
- Is congestion localised or generalised? Localised causes include episcleritis or phlycten.
- If generalised congestion is present, is it conjunctival or circum-corneal (perilimbic)? Circumcorneal causes include corneal disease, iridocyclitis and acute glaucoma.
- Check the cornea by instilling fluorescein drops.
- Check the visual acuity. Reduced acuity suggests sight-threatening pathology.
- Check the pupil reflexes. An absent or sluggish response is sinister.
- Is the globe tender? This may be a sign of glaucoma.

Haemorrhage

The commonest type is a subconjunctival bleed from a small vessel. The posterior edge of the haemorrhage will be visible. It looks alarming but clears spontaneously with no adverse consequences. If it is recurrent, check for a bleeding diathesis and hypertension.

Retrobulbar haemorrhages are rare but potentially sight-threatening. They occur after surgery, trauma or head injuries, and with bleeding diatheses. The posterior edge of the bleed is not visible, and proptosis and restricted eye movements may be noted.

Conjunctivitis

This is generally bilateral, so be alert for the unilateral red eye. Causes include allergy and viral and bacterial infections. Allergic and viral subtypes are normally self-limiting, but bacterial infection (indicated by muco-purulent discharge with possible lymphadenopathy) requires treatment with topical antibiotics.

Corneal disease

Corneal ulceration leads to a breach in the epithelium. Fluorescein staining will demonstrate these lesions glowing green under blue light. Causes include a foreign body or trauma from contact lens use.

Keratitis is inflammation of the cornea. Ulcerative keratitis is inflammation of the cornea associated with corneal ulceration. This is an ophthalmological emergency and requires immediate treatment. Causes include infection (bacterial, viral, fungal and protozoan) and vasculitis. Treatment will depend on the cause.

Iridocyclitis

This is often bilateral and presents with photophobia, acute pain, blurred vision, increased lacrimation and a small pupil (due to spasm of the iris). The condition is usually immune mediated, and there is a strong association with connective tissue disorders and joint disease. Recurrent attacks may occur and predipose the patient to glaucoma. The condition should be managed by an ophthalmologist. Treatment includes topical steroid drops and mydriatics (pupil dilation helps to prevent the formation of adhesions between the lens and the iris).

Acute glaucoma

This condition is most common in middle-aged or elderly, long-sighted patients with shallow anterior chambers. It arises when there is a block to the drainage of aqueous humour from the anterior chamber via the canal of Schlemm, most commonly in response to anticholinergic drugs or at night when the pupil dilates. This causes a rise in intra-ocular pressure.

Patients complain of a painful, red eye and blurred vision. They may be systemically unwell with nausea and vomiting. The eye is hard and tender, and the pupil may be fixed and dilated.

Treatment consists of reducing the intra-ocular pressure. Acetazolamide reduces the formation of aqueous humour. Constriction of the pupil with pilocarpine may open up the blocked drainage route. Surgical (or laser) iridectomy is performed once the pressure has been reduced (or rarely as an emergency). This involves removal of a small portion of the iris to ensure free circulation of aqueous humour.

Optic neuritis

This is inflammation of the optic nerve, and it may be visible as swelling of the disc. There is a reduction in visual acuity, patients notice problems with colour vision and eye movements may be painful. There is an afferent pupil defect (loss of direct response). Optic neuritis is rarely caused by diabetes or unusual infections such as syphilis. More commonly it may be the first manifestation of multiple sclerosis (MS).

Treatment with high-dose intravenous steroids for 3 days followed by oral steroids reduces the rate of development of MS over the next 2 years. There is also evidence that β-interferon given early reduces the likelihood of MS developing.

Further reading

- Foroozan R, Buono LM, Savino PJ and Sergott RC (2002) Acute demyelinating optic neuritis. *Curr Opin Ophthalmol.* **13**: 375–80.
- Warrell D, Cox TM, Firth JD and Benz EJ (2003) *Oxford Textbook of Medicine* (4e). Oxford University Press, Oxford.

Sudden loss of vision

Aetiology

The main causes of sudden loss of vision are summarised in Table 25.

Table 25   Causes of painless and painful loss of vision

Painless loss of vision	Painful loss of vision
Vascular occlusion	Corneal disease*
Retinal detachment	Iridocyclitis*
Vitreous haemorrhage	Acute angle-closure glaucoma*
Ischaemic optic neuropathy	Optic neuritis*
Age-related macular degeneration (wet variety)	

* see pp. 177–8.

Central retinal artery occlusion

Occlusion is normally due to emboli arising from atheromatous plaques or calcified heart valves. These may be visible at fundoscopy. Visual loss is rapid. The retina swells and becomes opaque with a 'cherry-red' spot visible at the fovea due to the intact choroidal circulation. If much of the retina is infarcted, there is loss of the direct pupil light reflex (afferent defect).

If the patient is seen within 1 hour it may be worth applying firm pressure to the globe, as this may help to dislodge the embolus into a peripheral vessel. Further management should include a carotid artery Doppler examination to assess the possible benefits of surgery. Risk factors such as hypertension, diabetes, hypercholesterolaemia, smoking and obesity should be managed, and treatment with aspirin should be commenced.

Central retinal vein occlusion

Risk factors include increasing age, chronic simple glaucoma, arterio-sclerosis, hypertension and polycythaemia. This condition is more common than arterial occlusion, and symptoms develop less abruptly. Patients often wake with blurred vision, and fundoscopy reveals a characteristic 'blood-storm' appearance. The prognosis is variable, with possible improvement over the next year, but macular oedema may lead to permanent central visual impairment. Retinal ischaemia may lead to new vessel formation, which may be controlled by laser photocoagulation. Risk factors should be minimised in order to prevent occlusion in the other eye. The benefits of long-term aspirin are unproven.

Retinal detachment

This may be idiopathic, secondary to an intra-ocular problem (e.g. vitreous bands), or it may occur after trauma (e.g. cataract surgery). There is also an association with myopia. Around 50% of patients will have warning signs such as light flashes or floaters (due to over-stimulation of the retina or bleeding within the eye). Patients describe the actual detachment as like 'a curtain coming down'. The macula may also become detached, leading to central visual loss. Field defects will be detected and there may be a decrease in visual acuity. Fundoscopy may reveal a grey retina that is ballooning forward. Urgent specialist referral is required, as surgery may help to secure the retina, although if the macula is affected, vision generally remains poor.

Vitreous haemorrhage

This is most common in patients with new vessel formation in the eye (e.g. in diabetes, sickle-cell disease, retinal vein occlusion or retinal detachment). It may also occur in patients with a bleeding diathesis. If the bleed is very large, the red reflex will be lost and it will be difficult to visualise the fundus. The haemorrhage will normally be absorbed spontaneously, but if it is still present after 3 months, vitrectomy may be required. The eyes should be reviewed regularly and photocoagulation of new vessels performed.

Ischaemic optic neuropathy

Ischaemia occurs as a result of occlusion of the posterior ciliary arteries by either arteriosclerosis or inflammation. One cause of local inflammation is temporal arteritis, a disorder associated with polymyalgia rheumatica. Symptoms include pain on chewing, scalp tenderness and general malaise. The ESR is elevated, and temporal artery biopsy may identify arteritis. Prompt treatment with high-dose oral steroids is required to prevent loss of vision in the other eye.

Age-related macular degeneration

This is the commonest cause of registered blindness in the UK. There are two subtypes, namely dry and wet age-related macular degeneration (AMD). Dry AMD is generally a slow process, whereas wet AMD may cause rapid loss of vision. Wet AMD is characterised by new vessel formation, haemorrhages and exudates. In some patients, photodynamic therapy may help to prevent leakage from the new vessels and thus avoid further visual loss.

Further reading

- Warrell D, Cox TM, Firth JD and Benz EJ (2003) *Oxford Textbook of Medicine* (4e). Oxford University Press, Oxford.
- Beatty S and Au Eong KG (2000) Acute occlusion of the retinal arteries: current concepts and recent advances in diagnosis and management. *J Accid Emerg Med.* **17**: 324–9.
- National Institute for Clinical Excellence (2003) *Macular Degeneration (Age-Related): photodynamic therapy*. National Institute for Clinical Excellence, London; www.nicc.org.uk

Maxillofacial trauma

Fractures of the facial skeleton are relatively common, especially after sporting injuries, road traffic accidents and assaults. They may be life-threatening due to associated airway obstruction, particularly in the case of middle-third and multiple mandibular fractures. In addition, depending on the mechanism of injury, cervical spine fractures may need to be excluded.

Examination

- Inspect the face from the front, the side and above. Look for:
  - asymmetry of the facial bones
  - flattening of the cheekbones
  - nasal deviation
  - uneven pupillary levels (due to orbital floor fractures)
  - subconjunctival haemorrhage without a posterior border (possible orbital wall fracture).
- Carefully feel along the contour of the facial bones. Surgical emphysema may suggest a fracture through a sinus.
- Check the range of eye movements, as the extra-ocular muscle attachments may be disrupted by orbital wall fractures.
- Check the patient's visual acuity.
- Examine the dental occlusion and ask the patient whether the teeth bite together normally. Check for any loose or missing teeth.
- Check the range of mandibular movements.
- Measure the intercanthal distance. If it is more than 3.5 cm, a naso-ethmoidal fracture should be suspected.
- Check for sensory abnormalities.

Radiology

- Particular views may be requested to help to identify specific fractures (e.g. orthopantogram for suspected mandibular fractures).
- Carefully trace the contour of the bones and compare it with the other side.
- Inspect the sinuses for asymmetry (opacities or fluid levels can help to identify a fracture).
- A chest X-ray may be required if there are missing teeth, crowns or dentures.

Management of the airway

Certain patterns of injury may compromise the airway and require immediate management.

- Posterior displacement of a fractured maxilla may block the naso-pharynx. This should be managed by placing two fingers above and behind the soft palate and gently drawing the maxilla forward.
- Bilateral mandibular fractures may cause posterior displacement of the tongue, blocking the oropharynx. The tongue may be drawn forward by placing a large traction suture in the anterior portion or grasping with a towel clip.
- Foreign bodies (e.g. teeth, dentures, bone, vomitus) may block the airway. Clear the oral cavity with a lateral finger sweep and suction.
- Bleeding may also obstruct the airway. Apply pressure or pack any open wounds. Nasal packing may also be required.
- Trauma to the larynx or trachea may cause severe oedema.
  - The history may be suggestive (e.g. blunt trauma caused by impact with a steering wheel).
  - Examination findings may include swelling, dyspnoea, altered voice, frothy haemorrhage or surgical emphysema.
  - High-dose intravenous steroids may enable endotracheal intubation.
  - A surgical airway (e.g. tracheostomy) may be needed if airway obstruction is complete.

Management of facial injuries

- Fractures of the mandible:
  - a fracture on one side of the mandible is often accompanied by a fracture on the other side in a different position
  - undisplaced fractures often do not require treatment. Displaced fractures will need fixation (e.g. by wiring teeth together or by direct wiring of bone)
  - any fracture that passes through a tooth socket requires antibiotics.
- Fractures of the middle third of the face:
  - all patients with these fractures require referral to the maxillo-facial surgeons
  - advise the patient not to blow their nose, and prescribe prophylactic antibiotics
  - ensure that tetanus prophylaxis is up to date.

- Facial lacerations should be cleaned but may require formal debridement. Do not close them, as they may provide access for assessing a fracture.
- Ensure that the patient receives adequate analgesia.

Further reading

- Hutchinson I and Hardee P (2000) Maxillofacial injuries. In: P Driscoll, D Skinner and R Earlam (eds) *ABC of Major Trauma* (3e). BMJ Books, London.
- Burkitt G and Quick CRG (eds) (2001) *Essential Surgery: problems, diagnosis and management* (3e). Churchill Livingstone, Edinburgh.

Epistaxis

This is a very common condition, with up to 60% of the population experiencing at least one episode in their lifetime, and 6% requesting medical assistance.

Anatomy

- The nasopharynx has a rich and superficial blood supply (one of its main functions is to warm and humidify air as it enters the respiratory tract).
- The majority (80%) of nosebleeds are anterior in origin and occur at an anastomosis on the lower part of the anterior nasal septum called Little's area. Branches of the external carotid artery supply this area.
- Posterior bleeding mainly arises from the posterior septal nasal artery.

Aetiology

- The majority of cases are idiopathic.
- Secondary causes include the following:
  - nasal trauma (e.g. picking nose, facial trauma, foreign body)
  - local nasal inflammation (e.g. due to allergic rhinitis, infection)
  - blood vessel abnormality
  - blood dyscrasias (e.g. thrombocytopenia, haemophilia)
  - neoplasia
  - drugs (e.g. cocaine, topical decongestants, warfarin)
  - hypertension.

Management

- If profuse bleeding is present, assess ABC and resuscitate as necessary.
- Minor bleeds may often be controlled by applying digital pressure over the soft cartilaginous portion of the nose for 10 minutes. Placing an icepack over the dorsum of the bridge of the nose may also be helpful. The patient should be asked to lean forward in order to reduce the risk of swallowing blood (this causes nausea).
- If this fails, cautery (e.g. with a silver nitrate stick) is the next step.
  - Prepare the nose by applying a local anaesthetic and vasoconstrictor (e.g. lidocaine with adrenaline) to the anterior nasal cavity, either by spraying or on a piece of cotton wool.
  - Ensure that you have a good light source (e.g. headlamp or otoscope).

- – Identify any prominent or bleeding vessels.
- – Apply the cautery stick to the vessel for approximately 10 seconds.
- – Do not cauterise both sides of the septum at the same time, as this increases the risk of necrosis and septal perforation.
- If bleeding continues, an anterior nasal pack should be sited.
  - – Nasal tampons may be applied horizontally along the floor of the nasopharynx. If these are not available, the cavity may be packed with ribbon gauze.
  - – If bleeding continues, bilateral packing may help to increase pressure over the septum, thereby reducing bleeding.
  - – Packs are often left *in situ* for 24–72 hours.
  - – Patients with packing *in situ* should be admitted to the ward due to the risk of airway obstruction. Antibiotics may also need to be commenced to reduce the risk of toxic shock syndrome.
- Posterior packing may be required for bleeding from the posterior nasal cavity. A number of commercial packs are available, but Foley catheters are commonly used.
  - – The catheter is inserted through the nostril and advanced until the tip is seen in the oropharynx.
  - – The balloon is inflated with 3–4 ml of water.
  - – The catheter is then pulled forward until it occludes the bleeding.
  - – The anterior nasal cavity is also packed (as described above).
- If bleeding continues despite conservative measures, surgical intervention may be necessary. This may involve any of the following:
  - – diathermy of the bleeding point under general anaesthetic
  - – septal surgery
  - – arterial ligation
  - – angiographic embolisation is also performed in some centres.
- All patients who are admitted to the ward should have blood taken for an FBC and group and save. Clotting studies should be requested for patients who are on anticoagulants or in whom a bleeding diathesis is suspected.

Further reading

- Pope LER and Hobbs CGL (2005) Epistaxis: an update on current management. *Postgrad Med J.* **81**: 309–14.
- Leong SCL, Roe RJ and Karkanevatos A (2005) No-frills management of epistaxis. *Emerg Med J.* **22**: 470–2.
- Majid AM and Kingsnorth AN (eds) (1998) *Fundamentals of Surgical Practice.* Greenwich Medical Media Ltd, London.

14 Paediatrics

Stridor

Differential diagnosis

- Croup.
- Foreign body.
- Acute epiglottitis.
- Smoke inhalation.
- Glandular fever.
- Bacterial tracheitis.
- Mediastinal tumour.
- Diphtheria.
- Laryngomalacia.
- Retropharyngeal abscess.
- Angioneurotic oedema.
- Tetany.

History

- Speed of onset of symptoms.
- Recent cough or cold.
- Possible foreign body inhalation.
- Is the child able to eat and drink?
- Are immunisations up to date?
- History of atopy or food allergy.

Examination

- General examination. Is the child ill? Can they speak? Are there any signs of a cold? What is their conscious level? Is fever present?
- Respiratory examination – assess the severity of stridor, the respiratory rate and the presence of cyanosis. Look for evidence of respiratory

distress (use of accessory muscles, chest wall recession and nasal flaring).
● Examination of the mouth – you can look inside if the child opens their mouth voluntarily. Do not use a spatula, as this may precipitate respiratory arrest.

Table 26   Characteristic features of epiglottitis and croup

Epiglottitis	Croup
Rapid onset	Slow onset
Severe stridor	Severe stridor is less common
Drooling saliva	No drooling
Weak voice	Hoarse voice or barking cough
May occur at any time	More common in evening or at night
Septicaemic	Normally systemically well (or mild pyrexia)

Investigations
● Chest X-ray: may identify a radiolucent foreign body.
● A full blood count is needed to help to distinguish between viral and bacterial infection.
● Blood cultures.

Management
This will depend on the cause of the stridor.

Croup
Croup most commonly occurs in children between the ages of 6 months and 3 years, but can also occur in children as young as 3 months and as old as 12–15 years. Around 75% of cases are caused by the parainfluenza virus. The symptoms of croup generally settle spontaneously within 48 hours, and most cases are managed at home.

A single oral dose of dexamethasone (0.15 mg/kg) has been shown to significantly reduce the proportion of children who require additional medical attention for mild croup symptoms. In more severe cases, nebulised budesonide has been found to be helpful, and it also reduces the need for epinephrine treatment in children with moderate to severe croup. Nebulised epinephrine is also of proven benefit. Antibiotics are not given.

Epiglottitis

Infection with *Haemophilus influenzae* causes rapid and intense swelling of the epiglottis and surrounding tissues. The condition is much less common than croup, and its incidence in children has decreased since the introduction of Hib (*Haemophilus influenzae* type b) vaccination to the paediatric schedule. It is an ENT emergency, as airway obstruction may occur suddenly.

Allow the child to adopt a comfortable position (normally upright with the neck extended) and give them oxygen. Avoid frightening the child further or examining the throat, as this may precipitate acute obstruction. Intravenous antibiotics (cephalosporin) should be given and elective intubation considered. Only a very experienced anaesthetist should perform the intubation. In an emergency, nebulised adrenaline may buy some time. Needle cricothyroidotomy may be required.

Further reading

- Denny F, Murphy TF, Clyde WA Jr *et al.* (1983) Croup: an 11-year study in a pediatric practice. *Pediatrics.* **71:** 871–6.
- Geelhoed GC, Turner J and Macdonald WB (1996) Efficacy of a small single dose of oral dexamethasone for outpatient croup: a double-blind placebo-controlled clinical trial. *BMJ.* **313:** 140–2.
- Ausejo M, Saenz A, Pham B *et al.* (2003) Glucocorticoids for croup. In: *The Cochrane Library. Issue 4.* Update Software, Oxford.
- Kristjansson S, Berg-Kelly K and Winso E (1994) Inhalation of racemic epinephrine in the treatment of mild and moderately severe croup. Clinical symptom score and oxygen saturation measurements for evaluation of treatment effects. *Acta Paediatr.* **83:** 1156–60.

Febrile convulsions

Febrile convulsions are acute seizures associated with fever that occur in children aged 6 months to 6 years, usually in response to a viral stimulus. There appears to be a genetic predisposition, as 50% of affected children have a positive family history. Febrile convulsions are common, affecting 3% of all children under the age of 6 years. Most febrile convulsions are of short duration (less than 5 minutes) and take the form of generalised tonic–clonic seizures.

Aetiology

Within the brain there are convulsant and anticonvulsant systems that vary with age. It is postulated that the balance of these systems changes, so that children who present with febrile convulsions have a lowered seizure threshold, which will improve with age.

History

- How long did the seizure last?
- Was it focal or generalised?
- Has it occurred before?
- What is the previous developmental history of the child?
- Is there a family history of epilepsy or febrile convulsions?

Examination

- Look for the cause of the fever.
- Do not forget to examine the ears and throat.
- Perform a thorough neurological examination and look for evidence of meningitis.

Investigations

These may not be necessary if the fit was of short duration, an obvious source of infection was found, and the child has had previous febrile convulsions. In children presenting with their first febrile convulsion, consider the following:

- FBC
- U&Es and glucose
- urinalysis
- chest X-ray

- lumbar puncture – particularly in children aged less than 18 months, as the signs of meningitis may be fairly non-specific in this age group.

Management

- Cool the child by removing their clothing, tepid bathing and administering antipyretics (e.g. paracetamol or ibuprofen).
- Fitting children should be given oxygen and the airway should be secured.
- Most seizures are of short duration and do not require drug therapy. However, any seizure that lasts for longer than 10 minutes should be actively treated with either rectal or intravenous diazepam.
- Admit the child if any of the following circumstances occur:
  - age less than 18 months
  - first febrile convulsion
  - serious infection (e.g. pneumonia)
  - pyrexia of unknown cause
  - prolonged seizure
  - parental anxiety.
- When the child is discharged, the parents should be advised about cooling measures and the risk of future seizures.
- If a child has recurrent febrile convulsions, rectal diazepam may be offered for the parents to administer themselves. This may be used either to terminate seizures that last longer than 5–10 minutes, or as prophylaxis in any febrile illness.
- Only a few children require continuous prophylaxis with anti-epileptic medication (e.g. those with recurrent prolonged seizures).

Prognosis

- Around 30–40% of children will have a further febrile convulsion.
- Only 1–2% will develop epilepsy.
- Epilepsy is more common in children with:
  - a first febrile convulsion before the age of 12 months
  - a prolonged seizure (lasting more than 30 minutes)
  - a complex initial seizure with neurological signs
  - more than three febrile convulsions.

Further reading

- McIntosh N, Helms PJ and Smyth R (eds) (2003) *Forfar and Arneil's Textbook of Paediatrics* (6e). Churchill Livingstone, Edinburgh.
- Hull D and Johnston D (1999) *Essential Paediatrics* (4e). Churchill Livingstone, Edinburgh.

Pyloric stenosis

This is the condition that most commonly requires surgery in infants, and it affects approximately 1 in every 300 children. The underlying pathology is hypertrophy of the circular fibres of the pylorus muscle, leading to gastric outlet obstruction. There is a multi-factorial mode of inheritance, with 20% of affected children having a positive family history.

Clinical features

Pyloric stenosis typically affects male (80% of cases) firstborn children. The main symptom is effortless vomiting which begins between the ages of 3 and 6 weeks. This becomes progressively more severe until it occurs after every feed and may be described as projectile. The vomitus usually contains curdled milk and gastric juices, but no bile, as the obstruction is proximal to the second part of the duodenum where the common bile duct drains into the gastrointestinal tract. In advanced cases, coffee-ground vomitus may be seen due to secondary gastritis.

Children with this condition are typically enthusiastic feeders (because they feel hungry). However, with time they will become dehydrated, which makes them listless and lethargic. They will fail to thrive, and in severe cases they may actually lose weight.

Pyloric stenosis is generally diagnosed clinically. The child may show signs of dehydration, and visible gastric peristalsis may be seen. The hypertrophied pyloric muscle (also known as the pyloric 'tumour') may be palpable in the epigastrium or right upper quadrant of the abdomen (examine from the left side with the left hand). The 'tumour' is the size of an olive, but may be difficult to locate due to the mobility of the pylorus.

Investigations

- Abdominal ultrasound examination can help to identify the pyloric tumour if it proves difficult to palpate.
- Electrolytes – in severe cases a metabolic alkalosis will be seen and there may be significant hyponatraemia, hypokalaemia and hypochloraemia.

Management

- It is important that the child is fully resuscitated before being taken to theatre. They will require intravenous fluids and monitoring of their fluid balance. It may take up to 24 hours to correct the associated electrolyte abnormalities.

- Once the child has been adequately resuscitated they will undergo a Ramstedt's pyloromyotomy, in which the circular muscle of the pylorus is divided down to the mucosa in order to relieve the obstruction.

Further reading

- McIntosh N, Helms PJ and Smyth R (eds) (2003) *Forfar and Arneil's Textbook of Paediatrics* (6e). Churchill Livingstone, Edinburgh.
- Hernanz-Schulman M (2003) Infantile hypertrophic pyloric stenosis. *Radiology.* **227**: 319–31.

Non-accidental injury

A child may be considered to be abused if he or she is treated by an adult (or another child) in a way that is unacceptable in a given culture at a given time. In 1962, a landmark paper was published which described the battered baby syndrome. Since that time, healthcare professionals have become increasingly skilled at detecting children who are being abused. However, a number of high-profile cases, such as that of Victoria Climbie, who died in 2000 with 128 separate injuries after months of systematic abuse, have highlighted the need for increased vigilance and a low threshold of suspicion.

History

- Full details of the incident that caused the injury should be obtained from the caregivers. An independent history from the child may also be useful.
- The child's personal history should include development and performance at school/nursery.
- Past illnesses and attendance at hospital, including history of previous injuries.
- Immunisations, drug history and allergies.
- Family history should include illnesses affecting siblings and parents (particularly psychiatric illness), and specific enquiry about inherited skin or blood disorders.
- Social history should contain the details of all siblings and household contacts.
- Systematic enquiry should include questions on bed wetting, soiling and general behaviour.

Examination

A general examination should include observation of the child's affect and relationships, including the interactions between the child, the parents and others present, and any behavioural problems. In particular, look out for 'frozen watchfulness', in which the child has an impassive facial appearance but carefully tracks the examiner with their eyes.

The child should be completely undressed and all findings carefully recorded. Height, weight and head circumference should be measured and plotted on growth charts.

Patterns of injury

Bruises

- Bruises to the eyes, mouth and/or ears.
- Bruises of different ages in the same place.
- Outline bruises (prints of hand, belt, shoes).
- Bruises to non-mobile babies.

Burns

- Clearly demarcated burns to a limb and/or buttock may suggest immersion in hot water.
- Small round burns may be caused by cigarettes.

Scars

- Large numbers of different-aged scars of unusual shape.
- Scars which indicate that the child did not receive medical attention.

Fractures

- Multiple fractures, especially of the ribs.
- Spiral fractures of long bones (humerus/femur).
- Any fracture in a child under 1 year of age.
- Fractures at different stages of healing.
- Depressed skull fractures.

Shaking

- Any bruising on a young child, particularly on the trunk, arms or face.
- Facial petechiae (small blood spots).
- Retinal haemorrhages.

Other patterns of injury

- Torn frenulum of the upper lip (caused by force-feeding).
- Bite marks – those more than 3 cm in diameter are unlikely to have been made by a child.

Diagnostic indicators

- Delay in seeking help, or not seeking it at all.
- Vague explanations lacking in detail.
- History incompatible with injury or developmental age (e.g. head injury due to child rolling off sofa at age of 6 weeks).
- Story changes over time or with different informants.
- Unusual parental behaviour (e.g. parent more interested in their own feelings than concerned for the child, or leaving before a senior doctor arrives).

Management

Some doctors are worried about sharing information in child protection cases, due to the need to break confidentiality. However, the General Medical Council states that it is not only permissible but also the duty of the doctor to do so. Doctors may discuss their concerns with other members of the healthcare team, such as health visitors or nurses, or may consult the child protection register. In some cases children may be admitted to hospital for treatment of their injuries, or if it is felt that the child would be unsafe if they returned home. However, in most instances concerns about non-accidental injury should be reported to social services for further investigation. Lord Laming in his report on the Victoria Climbie case emphasised the need for individuals to own their concerns – the person who first has a concern has the responsibility to take it further, rather than to 'just pass it on to the health visitor'.

Further reading

- Kempe CH, Silverman FN, Steele BF, Droegemuller W and Silver HK (1962) The battered child syndrome. *JAMA*. **181:** 17–24.
- Advanced Life Support Group (2001) *Advanced Paediatric Life Support: the practical approach* (3e). BMJ Books, London.
- General Medical Council (2004) *Confidentiality: protecting and providing information*. General Medical Council, London.
- Lord Laming/Great Britain Home Office (2003) *The Victoria Climbie Inquiry Report*. The Stationery Office, London; www.victoria-climbie-inquiry.org.uk

Paediatric trauma and resuscitation

Causes of cardiorespiratory arrest

Respiratory arrest commonly precedes cardiorespiratory arrest. It has a variety of underlying causes, including infections, foreign bodies, asthma and neurological dysfunction (e.g. head injury, drugs and fits). Cardiac arrests are uncommon and have a poor prognosis. They are most commonly related to underlying congenital cardiac disease or hypoxia following a respiratory arrest.

Differences between children and adults

- Airway:
  - young children have large heads and short necks, which tends to cause neck flexion and therefore narrowing of the airway.
- Breathing:
  - children under 6 months of age are obligate nasal breathers
  - the airways are relatively small and are therefore more easily obstructed
  - it is important to assess the effort of breathing. This includes respiratory rate, chest wall recession and grunting. In infants, look for head bobbing and flaring of the nostrils.
- Circulation:
  - severe hypoxia causes bradycardia, which is a pre-terminal sign
  - hypotension is a late and pre-terminal sign.
- Body surface area:
  - children's small size means that they have a high body surface area:weight ratio. This makes them more susceptible to hypothermia.

Table 27   Normal values for respiratory rate and heart rate in children

Age (years)	Respiratory rate (breaths/min)	Heart rate (beats/min)
< 1	30–40	110–160
1–2	25–35	100–150
2–5	25–30	95–140
5–12	20–25	80–120
> 12	15–20	60–100

Basic life support

There are some major differences between paediatric and adult basic life support. These are summarised in the algorithm below.

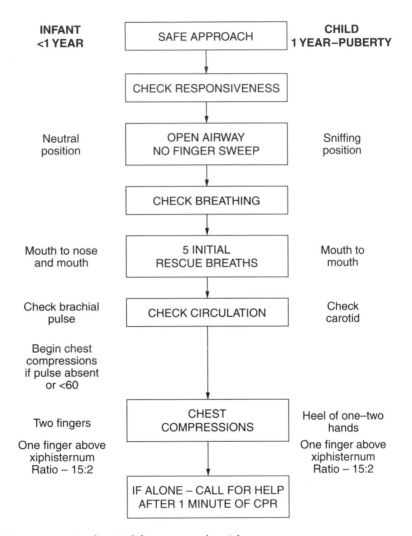

Figure 15 Paediatric life support algorithm

Advanced life support

Follow the standard protocols, bearing in mind the following points.

- Airway:
  - use a straight-blade laryngoscope and uncuffed endotracheal tube in children up to the age of 10 years.
- Breathing:
  - children are prone to swallowing air and vomiting, so site a nasogastric tube early to deflate the stomach.
- Circulation:
  - if intravenous access is not available, use the intra-osseous route.
- Asystole is the commonest rhythm seen at arrest.
- Drugs during CPR:
  - give adrenaline every 3–5 minutes. The dose is 10 mcg/kg on each occasion
  - consider the use of atropine when a bradycardia is unresponsive to improved ventilation and circulatory support. The dose is 20 mcg/kg (minimum dose 100 mcg, maximum 600 mcg)
  - give magnesium sulphate to children with documented hypo-magnesemia or 'torsades de pointes'. Administer by intravenous infusion over several minutes at a dose of 25–50 mg/kg (maximum 2 g).
- Ventricular fibrillation (VF) is uncommon:
  - give adrenaline (10 mcg/kg) before the third shock and subsequently before alternate shocks (approximately every 3–5 minutes)
  - in shock resistant VF consider the use of amiodarone 5 mg/kg before the fourth shock.

Table 28   Essential formulae

Weight	$(age + 4) \times 2$
Fluids	20 ml/kg
DC shocks	4 J/kg for the first and subsequent shocks
Endotracheal tube	$(Age/4) + 4$
Initial adrenaline dose (10 mcg/kg)	0.1 ml/kg of 1:10 000 solution

Paediatric trauma

- Follow the usual ABC principles of advanced trauma life support.
- Children have relatively elastic tissues, so the force of an impact may be dissipated away from the site of injury.
- Pelvic bone and rib fractures suggest high-force trauma, as these bones are more elastic in children.

- In young children the total circulating blood volume is small, so relatively small amounts of blood loss may be significant.
- Administer 10 ml/kg boluses of crystalloid for hypotension, with frequent reassessment.
- Urgent surgical review is indicated if a child has not stabilised after 20 ml/kg of crystalloid has been administered.
- Once 40 ml/kg has been given, blood should be used for any further fluid replacement.

Further reading

- Mackway-Jones K *et al.* (eds) (2005) *Advanced Paediatric Life Support: the practical approach* (4e). BMJ Books, London.
- Resuscitation Council (UK) (2005) *Paediatric Advanced Life Support*. Resuscitation Council (UK), London; www.resus.org.uk/pages/pals.pdf
- Resuscitation Council (UK) (2005) *Paediatric Basic Life Support*. Resuscitation Council (UK), London; www.resus.org.uk/pages/pbls.pdf

15 Obstetrics/ gynaecology

Ectopic pregnancy

An ectopic pregnancy is any pregnancy that implants outside the uterine cavity. The majority (95%) will implant within the Fallopian tube, but other sites include the abdomen, ovary and cervix. The incidence of ectopic pregnancy in the UK is 11 in 1000 pregnancies, and nearly 32 000 ectopic pregnancies were diagnosed in the UK during the 3-year period from 1997 to 1999.

Predisposing factors

- Pelvic inflammatory disease.
- Previous tubal pregnancy.
- Tubal surgery (e.g. sterilisation).
- Tubal disease (e.g. endometriosis).
- Infertility – there is an increased risk of ectopic pregnancy in women who have received treatment for subfertility. This may be due to pre-existing tubal disease.
- Intrauterine devices – although the total number of ectopic pregnancies is reduced in this group of women, there is an increased ratio of ectopic to intrauterine pregnancies.
- The progesterone-only pill and the 'morning-after pill' – these have a similar effect to intrauterine devices.

Clinical features

The classic triad of symptoms is amenorrhoea, abdominal pain and vaginal bleeding. The abdominal pain typically precedes the bleeding and is initially unilateral. The pain then becomes generalised due to blood loss into the peritoneal cavity; and there may be referred shoulder-tip pain due to diaphragmatic irritation. Patients may show signs of shock and peritonism.

Patients may also present subacutely with a short period of amenor-rhoea and intermittent attacks of recurrent vaginal bleeding or abdominal pain. An adnexal mass may be palpable on vaginal examination. Up to 25% of women will not have amenorrhoea or vaginal bleeding. A high index of suspicion is required in all women of childbearing age who present with any combination of the above symptoms.

Investigations

In the acutely shocked patient, surgical management should not be delayed by investigations. In other patients the following tests may be useful:

- pregnancy test – positive in 95% of ectopic pregnancies
- ultrasound examination – transvaginal ultrasound will detect early pregnancies from approximately 5 weeks' gestation. If no intrauterine pregnancy is detected, it may be possible to identify features of an ectopic pregnancy such as an extra-uterine embryo or sac, an adnexal mass or free fluid in the pouch of Douglas
- quantitative measurement of human chorionic gonadotropin (HCG) – problems arise in symptomatic women at very early gestations who have a positive pregnancy test but no features of either an intrauterine or extrauterine pregnancy on ultrasound examination. It may be useful to check serial serum HCG measurements. In viable intrauterine pregnancies, the hormone level should double over 48 hours, whereas a slowly rising or static HCG level suggests either an ectopic or a non-viable pregnancy. Intrauterine pregnancies should all be visible on vaginal ultrasound examination when the HCG level is > 2000 IU
- FBC and group and save.

Management

- Resuscitate shocked patients.
- Laparotomy should be performed in women who are haemodynam-ically unstable.
- Laparoscopy is the preferred approach for haemodynamically stable patients.
- Salpingotomy is the treatment of choice in patients with contralateral tubal disease. Compared with salpingectomy there is an increased risk of bleeding, persistent trophoblast and subsequent ectopic preg-nancy.

- Salpingectomy may be used in women who have a healthy contra-lateral tube or who have completed their families.
- Intramuscular methotrexate is an alternative treatment for early ectopic pregnancies.
- Expectant management may be an option in stable, asymptomatic women with an early ectopic pregnancy but falling HCG levels.
- Anti-D immunoglobulin should be administered to rhesus-negative women.

Further reading

- Bouyer J, Coste J, Fernandez H, Pouly JL and Job-Spira N (2002) Sites of ectopic pregnancy: a 10-year population-based study of 1800 cases. *Hum Reprod.* **17:** 3224–30.
- Tulandi T and Saleh A (1999) Surgical management of ectopic pregnancy. *Clin Obstet Gynecol.* **42:** 31–8.
- Royal College of Obstetricians and Gynaecologists (2004) *Clinical Green Top Guideline No. 21. The management of tubal pregnancy.* Royal College of Obstetricians and Gynaecologists, London; www. rcog.org.uk

Placenta praevia

Placenta praevia occurs when either the entire placenta or a part of it implants into the lower segment of the uterus. If the placenta encroaches on or covers the cervical os it is classified as a major placenta praevia. If it does not encroach on the os it is classified as a minor placenta praevia.

Risk factors

- High parity.
- Multiple pregnancy (large placental area).
- Rhesus disease.
- Previous myometrial damage (e.g. post curettage or Caesarean section).
- Placenta praevia in a previous pregnancy.

Clinical features

- Painless vaginal bleeding.
- Malpresentation of the fetus (e.g. high presenting part, breech or abnormal lie).
- Uterine hypotony.

Assessment

- The patient's haemodynamic condition, including pulse and blood pressure.
- Abdominal palpation – there is often a high presenting part with soft, atonic uterus.
- Cardiotopography to check fetal and uterine activity.
- Speculum examination should be performed to assess the amount and site of bleeding, liquor and cervical dilatation.
- If time permits, transvaginal ultrasound examination is the usual method of diagnosis. MRI scanning has been used in a number of trials, but is not performed routinely.
- *Do not perform a digital rectal examination until placenta praevia has been excluded.*

Management of minor haemorrhage

- Obtain IV access.
- Take blood for FBC, group and save, U&Es and clotting status.

- If the bleeding settles, assess the degree of placenta praevia. If a major placenta praevia is present, the patient will need to be admitted to hospital with blood cross-matched to await fetal maturity.
- Fetal growth and placental position should be assessed by ultrasound examination every 2 weeks.
- If a major degree of placenta praevia exists at 38 weeks' gestation, an elective Caesarean section should be performed.
- Women with minor degrees of placenta praevia may be allowed a trial of spontaneous labour.

Management of an active, significant bleed

- Obtain IV access.
- Take blood for FBC, group and save, U&Es and clotting status.
- If the estimated blood loss is greater than 300 ml, cross-match at least 2 units of blood.
- Begin IV fluid resuscitation while awaiting cross-matched blood if there is significant bleeding.
- If there is heavy bleeding, the patient should be examined by senior staff in theatre.
- If there is fetal distress, the case should be discussed with the consultant in charge and a decision made about possible delivery.
- The mode of delivery will depend on the clinical situation. However, a placenta encroaching within 2 cm of the internal os is a contra-indication to attempting vaginal delivery.
- Senior anaesthetists should be involved if a decision is made to perform emergency Caesarean section.

Complications

- These patients are at risk of postpartum haemorrhage, so senior staff should be involved and Syntocinon administered at the time of delivery.
- Be aware of the high risk of a morbidly adherent placenta in patients with placenta praevia and a previous Caesarean section scar.

Further reading

- Royal College of Obstetricians and Gynaecologists (2005) *Clinical Green Top Guideline No. 27. Placenta praevia and placenta praevia accreta: diagnosis and management.* Royal College of Obstetricians and Gynaecologists, London; www.rcog.org.uk

Placental abruption

This may be defined as haemorrhage resulting from premature separation of the placenta before delivery of the child. The aetiology of the condition is unknown.

Associated factors

- Hypertension.
- Pre-eclampsia.
- Smoking during pregnancy.
- Low socio-economic status.
- Previous placental abruption.
- Trauma.
- Male infant.
- Intrauterine growth retardation.

Clinical features

- Vaginal bleeding (although it is not present in all cases).
- Sudden onset of severe abdominal pain.
- Longitudinal lie.
- Fundal size may appear large for dates, with concealed haemorrhage (which occurs between the placenta and the uterine wall).
- Tense, hard uterus.
- Shocked patient.
- Patient may be in labour (precipitated by the placental abruption).
- Fetal hearts sounds may be absent.

Assessment

- Assess the patient's haemodynamic condition, including pulse and blood pressure.
- Abdominal palpation reveals a tense, tender uterus. It is often difficult to palpate the fetal parts.
- Cardiotopography to check fetal and uterine activity.

Management

- Obtain IV access.
- Take blood for FBC, U&Es, clotting status and cross-matching.

- Begin IV fluid resuscitation while awaiting cross-matched blood if there is significant bleeding.
- Call senior colleagues for help.
- Any significant placental abruption should be treated by delivering the fetus as soon as possible.

Complications

- Disseminated intravascular coagulation:
    - severe placental abruption leads to the release of thromboplastin into the maternal circulation, and may trigger this potentially fatal condition
    - patients should be managed in an ITU bed and will require infusion of fresh-frozen plasma, platelets and clotting factors.
- Postpartum haemorrhage.
- Renal tubular or cortical necrosis – this condition is increasingly rare but may require dialysis.
- Fetal death.

Further reading

- Symonds EM and Symonds IM (2003) *Essential Obstetrics and Gynaecology* (4e). Churchill Livingstone, Edinburgh.

Pre-eclampsia

Pre-eclampsia is characterised by raised blood pressure associated with proteinuria that develops after 20 weeks' gestation. It is a multi-system disease that may affect the liver, kidneys, coagulation and cardiovascular systems, and placental infarcts may also be seen. It is a major cause of maternal mortality (15–20% in western countries).

Definitions

- *Mild hypertension:* blood pressure of 140/90 mmHg on two occasions or an increase of 30 mmHg systolic or 15 mmHg diastolic from the time of booking.
- *Severe hypertension:* diastolic blood pressure greater than 110 mmHg on two occasions or greater than 120 mmHg on one occasion.
- *Proteinuria:* exceeding 0.3 g in 24 hours.

Aetiology

The exact aetiology remains unknown. However, an immunological basis is suspected due to the lower incidence of pre-eclampsia in consanguineous marriages, and its increased incidence in the first pregnancies of second marriages. Research into the condition has also demonstrated associations with systemic vascular resistance, enhanced platelet aggregation, activation of the coagulation system, and endothelial-cell dysfunction. Low-dose aspirin has been shown to be of some benefit to women who are at risk of early, severe pre-eclampsia.

Clinical features

- The patient is often asymptomatic until late in the disease process.
- Oedema – pedal oedema is particularly common in pregnancy, so is a fairly non-specific symptom. Hand and facial oedema may also be seen.
- Patients may complain of other symptoms, including frontal headaches, photophobia, diplopia or flashing lights. Epigastric pain accompanied by nausea or vomiting may signify severe pre-eclampsia and possibly imminent eclampsia.
- Examination findings may include oedema, epigastric or liver tenderness, hyperreflexia and clonus. The fundi should be examined for haemorrhages.

- The fundal height may be small for dates (pre-eclampsia is a common cause of intrauterine growth retardation).

Investigations

- Send an MSU to exclude infection.
- Twenty-four-hour protein collection.
- FBC, U&Es, urate, LFTs and group and save.
- Cardiotopography, umbilical artery Doppler and ultrasound examination to assess liquor volume/fetal size.

Management

This will depend on the severity of the hypertension, proteinuria and symptoms. Once assessed, mild cases may be managed in the community with daily checks by a midwife. More severe cases will require inpatient management.

- Blood pressure – severe hypertension (> 160/110 mmHg) requires treatment to reduce the risk of cerebrovascular haemorrhage. Drugs that may be used include hydralazine, nifedipine, beta-blockers and methyldopa.
- Magnesium sulphate therapy is used to prevent convulsions. It is indicated in women with neurological symptoms or signs, impaired liver function, marked renal impairment or coagulopathy.
- Fluid balance – pre-eclamptic patients may be hypoalbuminaemic, with increased capillary permeability. This predisposes to tissue oedema together with low plasma volumes. Patients require careful monitoring and judicious fluid administration to prevent pulmonary or cerebral oedema. CVP monitoring may be necessary.
- HELLP syndrome is characterised by haemolysis, elevated liver enzymes and low platelet levels. This is a variant of pre-eclampsia in which there is an increased rate of disseminated intravascular coagulation and placental abruption. Haematological advice must be sought to help to manage this condition.
- Give steroids to promote fetal respiratory maturity.
- It is important to recognise that pre-eclampsia does not improve and that delivery may be required to 'treat' the condition. The timing and method of delivery will depend on the severity of the condition, the gestational age and the state of the cervix.
- Women require continued monitoring after delivery, as there is a significant risk of eclamptic fits (50% of cases occur after delivery).

Blood pressure may remain raised and require continued treatment (normally with beta-blockers or nifedipine).

Eclampsia

- This is the onset of fits, in pregnancies complicated by pre-eclampsia, after 20 weeks' gestation.
- There is increased maternal mortality (due to cerebral haemorrhage) and fetal death.
- Basic management of the seizure includes opening the airway, administering oxygen and giving diazepam.
- The blood pressure must be controlled.
- Urgent delivery is a priority for both the fetus and the mother.

Further reading

- Sibai B, Dekker G and Kupferminc M (2005) Pre-eclampsia. *The Lancet*. **365**: 785–99.
- Symonds EM and Symonds IM (2003) *Essential Obstetrics and Gynaecology* (4e). Churchill Livingstone, Edinburgh.

Cord prolapse

Cord prolapse occurs when the umbilical cord lies in front of the presenting part after rupture of the membranes. The cord may prolapse into the vagina, or even beyond the introitus, and may be compressed by the presenting part. Cord presentation occurs when the cord is presenting but the forewaters are still intact.

Risk factors

- Breech presentation.
- High presenting part (e.g. secondary to placenta praevia or fibroids).
- Cephalo-pelvic disproportion.
- Transverse lie.
- Unstable lie.
- Polyhydramnios.

Diagnosis

- The condition is diagnosed by palpation of the cord in the vagina.
- The condition may be suspected if fetal heart rate decelerations or bradycardia are observed in any woman at risk of cord prolapse.

Management

- The person making the diagnosis must keep their hand in the vagina and attempt to prevent cord compression by the presenting part.
- The obstetric specialist registrar should be crash called.
- Move the woman into a position that will allow gravity to pull the presenting part away from the cord (e.g. on all fours or lying in the left lateral opposition with the head of the bed tilted down).
- Avoid handling the cord, in order to minimise spasm of the cord vessels.
- If the cord has prolapsed beyond the introitus, dehydration and spasm of the cord may occur. If possible, replace the cord within the vagina. If this is not possible, wrap the cord in a warm, sterile, damp cloth.
- If the cervix is fully dilated, an experienced obstetrician must decide whether instrumental vaginal delivery is possible. If it is not, the theatre team should be crash called for an immediate Caesarean section.
- A paediatrician must be present at the delivery.

- Blood should be taken for blood gas analysis post delivery.
- If the cord prolapse occurs outside hospital and the patient needs to be transported, a Foley catheter may be sited and 500 ml of saline infused into the bladder to keep the presenting part out of the pelvis in an attempt to prevent cord compression.

Prognosis

If the cord prolapse occurs in hospital and is rapidly dealt with, the outcome is normally good. There is a poorer prognosis if the cord prolapse occurs outside hospital.

Further reading

- Symonds EM and Symonds IM (2003) *Essential Obstetrics and Gynaecology* (4e). Churchill Livingstone, Edinburgh.
- Runnebaum IB and Katz M (1999) Intrauterine resuscitation by rapid bladder instillation in a case of occult prolapse of an excessively long umbilical cord. *Eur J Obstet Gynecol Reprod Biol.* 84: 101–2.
- Katz Z, Shoham Z, Lancet M *et al.* (1988) Management of labor with umbilical cord prolapse: a 5-year study. *Obstet Gynecol.* 72: 278–80.

Shoulder dystocia

Shoulder dystocia occurs when the head is delivered but the anterior shoulder is obstructed by the pubic symphysis. Rarely there is also obstruction of the descent of the posterior shoulder by the sacral promontory, so that both shoulders are arrested above the pelvic brim (bilateral shoulder dystocia).

Once the head has been delivered, oxygen delivery to the fetus is reduced, as the chest is compressed so effective breaths are not possible. In addition, uterine contraction occurs, leading to decreased blood flow. If there is no preceding hypoxia, hypoxic brain damage will occur after 4–5 minutes if the shoulders are not delivered.

Shoulder dystocia is a relatively common condition with a reported incidence ranging from 0.2% to 2% of all vaginal cephalic deliveries. It is therefore important that all professionals attending deliveries know how to manage the condition.

Table 29   Risk factors for shoulder dystocia

Antepartum	*Intrapartum*
Macrosomia (increased risk with increased birth weight)	Protracted or arrested cervical dilatation during first stage of labour
Infants of diabetic mothers (have an increased shoulder:head circumference ratio)	Protracted or arrested descent during second stage of labour
Postmaturity	Prolonged second stage of labour
Maternal obesity	
Previous infant > 4.5 kg	
Previous shoulder dystocia	

Management

- Call for help from senior colleagues (midwife, obstetrician, paediatrician and anaesthetist).
- Place the patient in the McRoberts' position. This is an exaggerated lithotomy position with abduction and acute flexion of the thighs. It causes superior rotation of the symphysis pubis and straightening of the lumbosacral angle, which may help to dislodge the anterior shoulder. It is generally atraumatic for both mother and child, and will resolve most mild to moderate cases of shoulder dystocia.
- Give analgesia and perform a large episiotomy.

- If this fails, ask an assistant to apply downward suprapubic pressure, which may help to rotate the shoulders from the narrow anterior–posterior diameter of the pelvis to the wider oblique diameter.
- Experienced obstetricians may attempt other manoeuvres such as Wood's screw manoeuvre (pushing the back of the posterior shoulder towards the chest of the fetus), which may rotate the shoulders to the oblique diameter. Attempts may also be made to deliver the posterior arm.
- Placing the woman in the 'all-fours' position has also been reported to be a successful technique. However, this may be difficult for a woman in the second stage of labour.
- As a last resort, cases of symphisotomy, clavicular fracture and cephalic replacement with Caesarean section have all been reported.
- Do not apply forceful traction to the fetal head. It will not help to resolve the situation, and it increases the likelihood of brachial plexus injury.

Complications

- Fetal complications are relatively common, and include clavicle fracture and brachial plexus injury, generally affecting the C5 and C6 nerve roots (Erb's palsy). Rarely, fetal asphyxia and permanent brain damage or death may occur.
- Maternal complications are more rare. Vaginal lacerations are more common, due to the manoeuvres employed, as is postpartum haemorrhage. Rarely uterine rupture may occur due to the application of excessive suprapubic pressure.

Further reading

- Baskett TF (2002) Shoulder dystocia. *Best Pract Res Clin Obstet Gynaecol.* **16:** 57–68.
- Gherman RB and Goodwin TM (1998) Shoulder dystocia. *Curr Opin Obstet Gynecol.* **10:** 459–63.

Postpartum haemorrhage

Definitions

- *Primary postpartum haemorrhage:* 500 ml blood loss from the genital tract within 24 hours of delivery.
- *Secondary postpartum haemorrhage:* excessive blood loss from the genital tract from 24 hours to 6 weeks after delivery.

Table 30   Predisposing factors for postpartum haemorrhage

Identified before labour	*Identified during labour*
Antepartum haemorrhage	Emergency Caesarean section
Previous postpartum haemorrhage	Elective Caesarean section
Multiple pregnancy	Retained placenta
Grand multiparity	Instrumental vaginal delivery
Pre-eclampsia	Prolonged labour (> 12 hours)
Coagulation disorders	

Causes

- Uterine atony – by far the commonest cause of postpartum haemorrhage.
- Retained products of conception.
- Cervical tears (most common at the 3 o'clock and 9 o'clock positions).
- Vaginal tears.
- Uterine rupture – rare, but more common in women with a previous Caesarean scar.

Prevention

- Identify risk factors and manage them appropriately (e.g. involve the haematologist at an early stage in the care of a woman with a coagulation disorder).
- Prophylactic oxytocic agents (e.g. oxytocin 10 IU) should be offered routinely in the management of the third stage of labour, as they reduce the risk of postpartum haemorrhage by about 60%.

Management

Primary postpartum haemorrhage (in shocked patient)

- Assessment.
  - Take blood for a full blood count, clotting status and cross-matching (2–6 units depending on the amount of blood loss and degree of shock).
  - Monitor the pulse and blood pressure.
  - Insert a urinary catheter to empty the bladder and accurately monitor urine output.
- Call for help.
  - Alert a senior midwife.
  - Alert a senior obstetrician.
  - Alert a senior anaesthetist.
  - Alert the haematologist and blood transfusion service.
  - Call porters for delivery of blood/specimens.
- Resuscitate.
  - Obtain IV access (14 G cannula × 2).
  - Head-down tilt.
  - Give oxygen by mask at a rate of 8 litres/minute.
  - Commence fluid resuscitation with crystalloid and colloid in turn while awaiting blood.
  - Transfuse blood as soon as possible.
  - If bleeding is unrelenting and the results of coagulation studies are still unavailable, consider the empirical use of fresh-frozen plasma and cryoprecipitate.
- Conservative management of bleeding.
  - Uterine compression ('rubbing up the fundus') to stimulate contractions.
  - Give Syntocinon, 10 units by slow IV injection.
  - Give a Syntocinon infusion.
  - Give carboprost (Hemabate), 0.25 mg IM (contraindicated in asthmatics). The dose may be repeated at a minimum of 15-minute intervals.
  - Bimanual compression of the uterus (one hand on the abdomen, and the other in the vagina pushing the uterus upwards).
  - Aortic compression (lift the uterus out of the pelvis and push it posteriorly against the aorta).

- Exclude other potential causes of postpartum haemorrhage.
  - Deliver the placenta (it may require manual removal under anaesthetic).
  - Identify and suture cervical/vaginal lacerations.
  - Explore the uterus (look for retained products of conception or evidence of uterine rupture).
- Surgical management. Options include the following:
  - uterine artery embolisation
  - bilateral ligation of uterine arteries
  - bilateral ligation of internal iliac arteries
  - haemostatic uterine suturing (e.g. B-Lynch)
  - hysterectomy.
- Consider transfer to an intensive-care unit.

Secondary postpartum haemorrhage

This is generally due to retained placental tissue or clot, and secondary infection is common. Bleeding may be light, in which case conservative management with oral antibiotics may be adequate. Uterine exploration will be necessary if bleeding is heavier, if retained products are identified on ultrasound examination or if the cervical os is open and the uterus is tender. The patient should have blood cross-matched and be given intravenous antibiotics pre-operatively. Uterine curettage must be very gentle, as the risks of perforation are higher in the puerperium.

Further reading

- Scottish Programme for Clinical Effectiveness in Reproductive Health (1998, updated 2002) *Scottish Obstetric Guidelines and Audit Project. The management of postpartum haemorrhage.* Scottish Programme for Clinical Effectiveness in Reproductive Health, Aberdeen; www.show.scot.nhs.uk/spcerh/

Toxic shock syndrome

Toxic shock syndrome (TSS) is a rare but life-threatening disease that is characterised by shock and multiple organ dysfunction. The syndrome was first described in 1978 in children, but became internationally recognised following an outbreak in women in the USA in 1980. Although TSS is more common in women, cases have also been reported in men and children. It most commonly affects young, healthy individuals aged 20–50 years.

Aetiology

Staphylococcus aureus is a bacterium that commonly colonises the skin and mucous membranes of humans. The commonest sites of carriage are the anterior nasopharynx, the vagina, the axillae and the perineum. TSS is caused by toxin-producing strains of *S. aureus*. The commonest TSS toxins are toxic shock syndrome toxin-1 (TSST-1; accounting for 75% of cases) and staphylococcal enterotoxin B (SEB; accounting for 20–25% of cases). It is believed that the clinical features of the syndrome are caused by massive release of cytokines in response to toxin activity.

Approximately half of all cases of TSS are associated with tampon use in menstruating women (numbers have fallen since the withdrawal of super-absorbent tampons). Non-menstrual cases tend to be associated with local or systemic *S. aureus* infections. Predisposing factors include the following:

- postpartum infections
- women using barrier contraceptives such as the diaphragm or contraceptive sponge
- sinusitis
- following nasal packing
- patients with burns
- post-operative skin infections
- osteomyelitis.

Diagnosis

Diagnosis of TSS is confirmed if all of the following five clinical criteria are fulfilled (a probable case fulfils four of the five criteria):

1 temperature ≥ 38.9°C (102°F)
2 hypotension or orthostatic syncope
3 a diffuse macular erythematous rash resembling sunburn

4 desquamation of skin, especially on the palms and soles, 1–2 weeks after the onset of illness

5 abnormalities in three or more of the following organ systems:

- gastrointestinal (vomiting or diarrhoea)
- muscular (myalgia or serum creatinine phosphokinase level at least twice the upper limit of normal)
- hepatic (serum bilirubin or transaminase levels at least twice the upper limit of normal)
- renal (urea or creatinine levels at least twice the upper limit of normal, or pyuria with > 5 white blood cells per high-power field in the absence of urinary tract infection)
- haematological (low platelet count, anaemia or disseminated intravascular coagulation)
- central nervous system (disorientation or altered consciousness with no focal findings)
- mucous membranes (conjunctival, oropharyngeal or vaginal hyperaemia).

In addition, there should be reasonable evidence of the absence of other illnesses (e.g. negative blood, throat and CSF cultures).

Management

- Identify and decontaminate the site of toxin production (e.g. remove tampon, drain or debride lesions and irrigate copiously). Recent surgical wounds should be explored and irrigated even if signs of inflammation are absent.
- Aggressive fluid resuscitation should be given to treat shock and prevent organ damage.
- Antibiotics should be given to eradicate *S. aureus* from the local site.
- Dialysis may be required in patients who develop renal failure.
- Transfer the patient to an intensive-care unit, as ventilatory and inotropic support is often required.

Prognosis

- The mortality rate is approximately 5%.
- TSS recurs in up to 40% of cases, and is linked to a failure to generate appropriate antibodies.

Streptococcal toxic shock syndrome

This syndrome was first described in 1987 in patients with group A streptococcal infection. The clinical features are similar to those of the staphylococcal toxic shock syndrome. Diagnostic criteria include isolation of group A streptococcus from a sterile body site, hypotension and multi-organ failure. Cutaneous signs may be subtle or absent. Streptococcal toxic shock syndrome is usually associated with necrotising fasciitis or myositis. It has a higher mortality rate than staphylococcal TSS.

Further reading

- Reingold AL, Hargrett N *et al.* (1982) Toxic shock syndrome surveillance in the United States, 1980 to 1981. *Ann Intern Med.* **96:** 875–80.
- Bisno AL and Stevens DL (1996) Streptococcal infections of the skin and soft tissues. *NEJM.* **334:** 240–45.

16 Psychiatric conditions

Acute psychosis: assessment

Acute psychosis is a psychiatric emergency. Patients may lack insight and there may be a high risk of self-injury or harm to others secondary to hallucinations or delusional thinking. A thorough assessment is necessary to identify the cause, especially in order to exclude any underlying organic conditions.

Setting
- Conduct the interview in a quiet, calm, private setting, preferably away from clinical areas.
- The majority of psychiatric patients are not violent. However, do not allow the need for privacy to compromise your personal safety.
- Make sure that other members of staff know where you are.
- Check with the staff to see if they are aware of any known risks.
- Ensure that you know how to call other staff should you need to (e.g. by using an alarm).
- Only take with you the equipment that you need for the assessment, and check that you have taken everything with you when you leave.
- Ensure that you sit between the door and the patient.

History
- Presenting complaint and history of present illness.
- Personal history – birth, infancy, childhood, employment and relationships.
- Family history – family structure, health and psychiatric history.
- Past medical history.
- Past psychiatric history.

- Drug history.
- Substance use history – alcohol, tobacco and illicit drugs.
- Social history – current circumstances, financial situation.
- Forensic history.
- Premorbid personality.

Risk assessment

- Risk to self – including past history of self-harm.
- Risk of neglect.
- Risk to others – previous incidents of violence, and any specific threats.
- Risk to children.

Physical examination

- This should focus on any conditions that may be associated with psychiatric disorders (e.g. thyroid disease, substance abuse/withdrawal, head injury, cerebrovascular disease and other intracranial pathology).
- Baseline observations (pulse, temperature, blood pressure and respiratory rate) should be completed.
- A careful neurological examination should be performed.
- Consider the use of a chaperone.

Investigation

- Blood glucose, electrolytes, TFTs, LFTs, and FBC.
- Urinalysis.
- A urine drug screen may be indicated.
- Further investigations (e.g. chest X-ray, ECG, CT scan of head) may be required if clinically indicated.

Differential diagnosis

- Schizophrenia.
- Mania.
- Depression with psychotic features.
- Puerperal illness.
- Drug induced, or linked to drug withdrawal.
- Other organic causes.

Box 1   Mental State Examination

Appearance and behaviour	• Clothing, make-up, cleanliness and tidiness • Posture and facial expression • Abnormal or spontaneous movements and mannerisms • Eye contact and rapport • Is the patient easily distracted or responding to hallucinations?
Speech	• Rate, volume, rhythm and spontaneity • Note any invented words (neologisms) or unusual phrases, puns or rhymes • Note any perseveration (repeating words or topics)
Mood	• Subjective and objective evaluation • Affect (or variability): normal, blunted or labile
Form of thought	• Loosening of associations (loss of links between topics) • Flight of ideas (moving rapidly from one idea to the next) • Thought block (e.g. 'my mind goes blank', 'my thoughts disappear')
Thought content	• Obsessional ideas (recurrent and intrusive, but recognised as the patient's own thoughts) • Ideas of reference (patient believes that others are talking about him) • Delusions (firmly held, false beliefs out of keeping with the patient's cultural norm and unshakeable by logical argument) • Passivity phenomena, including thought insertion, withdrawal and broadcast • Suicidal ideation and plans
Perceptions	• Illusions (misperceptions of external stimuli) • Hallucinations (perceptions in the absence of external stimuli); auditory hallucinations are most common with psychiatric disorder, hallucinations in other modalities may be associated with organic disorders
Cognition	• Conscious level • Orientation with regard to time, place and person • Memory • Attention and concentration • Ability to interpret instructions and perform tasks
Insight	• Patient's understanding of their condition • Patient's willingness to accept treatment

Further reading

- Gelder M *et al.* (eds) (2000) *New Oxford Textbook of Psychiatry*. Oxford University Press, Oxford.
- Royal College of Psychiatrists (1999) *Safety for Trainees in Psychiatry. Report of the Collegiate Trainees' Committee Working Party on the Safety of Trainees*. Royal College of Psychiatrists, London.
- Royal College of Psychiatrists (1996) *Assessment and Clinical Management of Risk of Harm to Other People. The Royal College of Psychiatrists Special Working Party on Clinical Assessment and Management of Risk*. Royal College of Psychiatrists, London.

Acute psychosis: management

Recognise the potential for violence

- The majority of psychiatric patients will not be violent, but when acutely psychotic they may lack insight and become easily frustrated.
- Risk factors include the following:
  - history of disturbed/violent behaviour
  - misuse of alcohol/illicit substances
  - command hallucinations
  - preoccupation with violent fantasies
  - delusions of control
  - agitation, excitement, overt hostility or suspicion.
- Look for the following warning signs:
  - increased restlessness or pacing
  - tense, angry facial expression
  - loud and high-pitched voice
  - pointing finger, erratic movements and invasion of personal space
  - verbal threats and gestures
  - refusal to communicate
  - unclear thought processes and poor concentration.
- If at any stage you are concerned about your physical safety, terminate the interview.
- If you are concerned about the possibility of potential violence, request the help of the on-call psychiatrist. They will be skilled in techniques of de-escalation and can advise on possible drug therapy.

De-escalation techniques

Verbal techniques

- Speak softly and calmly.
- Show that you are listening to the patient.
- Communicate clearly.
- Acknowledge the patient's concerns.
- Emphasise co-operation.
- Try to offer solutions.

Non-verbal techniques

- Avoid prolonged eye contact, which can be perceived as threatening.
- Adopt a distanced, neutral stance.
- Use open gestures, with the hands down.
- Sit down (if it is safe to do so).
- Move any audience away.

Rapid tranquillisation

If non-drug measures have been unsuccessful, drug therapy may be used to calm the patient and reduce the risk of violence to him- or herself or to others. It is important to avoid over-sedation – patients should be able to respond to communication throughout.

- Offer oral medication – short-acting benzodiazepine (e.g. lorazepam 2 mg) with or without an antipsychotic (e.g. haloperidol 2.5–5 mg).
- Consider intramuscular injection if:
  - oral therapy is refused or has failed
  - oral therapy is not indicated due to previous clinical response to oral medication.
- Consider IM lorazepam and haloperidol (dose according to *British National Formulary*).

Notes on prescribing rapid tranquillisation

- Lower doses are required in the elderly due to the higher risk of side-effects. Caution should also be exercised in patients with concomitant physical disorders.
- Benzodiazepines are the treatment of choice for patients who are already taking antipsychotics or who are antipsychotic naive.
- Use benzodiazepines with caution in patients with respiratory disease.
- The side-effects of benzodiazepines include loss of consciousness and respiratory depression. *Note*: there is a risk of cardiovascular system collapse when these drugs are prescribed with clozapine.
- Ensure that flumazenil is available when prescribing benzodiazepines.
- The side-effects of antipsychotics include loss of consciousness, cardiovascular/respiratory system collapse, seizures, dystonia, neuroleptic malignant syndrome and excessive sedation.
- When using haloperidol, procyclidine should be immediately available to reduce the risk of dystonia or other extrapyramidal side-effects.

Physical intervention

- Physical restraint should be avoided if at all possible.
- If physical intervention is necessary, it should be terminated as rapidly as possible.
- Restraint should only be practised by trained staff with a leader responsible for protecting and supporting the patient's head and neck.
- Physical restraint may be used to allow rapid tranquillisation to be administered and/or take effect.

The Mental Health Act (1983)

If patients refuse to be admitted to hospital and it is felt that they may present a danger to themselves or others, staff have emergency legal powers to detain them under the auspices of this Act.

Table 31   Mental Health Act (1983)

Section	Reason	Medical recommendation	Applicant	Duration
S2	Assessment and treatment	2 doctors, of whom 1 is approved (under S12 of Mental Health Act)	Relative or ASW	28 days
S3	Treatment	1 doctor	Relative or ASW	6 months
S4	Emergency admission	1 doctor	Relative or ASW	72 hours
S5 (2)	Inpatient emergency	1 doctor	–	72 hours
S5 (4)	Nurse's holding power	1 RMN	–	6 hours

Further reading

- National Institute for Clinical Excellence (2005) *CG25 Violence: quick reference guide.* National Institute for Clinical Excellence, London; www.nice.org.uk/pdf/cg025quickrefguide.pdf
- Gelder M *et al.* (eds) (2000*) New Oxford Textbook of Psychiatry.* Oxford University Press, Oxford.

Deliberate self-harm and suicide

Suicide may be defined as intentional self-inflicted death. The death rate from suicide and undetermined injury in England in 2002 was 8.9 per 100 000 population. This is equivalent to approximately 4500 suicides in England every year. Suicide is the commonest cause of death in men under 35 years of age. In 1999 the UK Government set a target of reducing the death rate from suicide and undetermined injury by at least one-fifth by the year 2010.

Aetiology

- *Mental disorders:* approximately 90% of people who commit suicide have a mental disorder at the time of death. The most common association is with severe depression (15% lifetime risk). Other mental disorders associated with suicide include alcohol abuse, personality disorder, schizophrenia, bipolar affective disorder and anorexia nervosa.
- *Copycat behaviour:* this may be seen, for example, after the suicide of a celebrity or occasionally within schools following the suicide of a pupil.

High-risk groups

- Men are much more likely to complete the act of suicide, as they use more violent and lethal methods. The suicide rate in young men is increasing.
- Elderly people (aged 65 years or over) represent 15% of the population but account for 20–25% of all completed suicides.
- People living alone or who are socially isolated.
- Unemployed individuals.
- Drug and alcohol abusers.
- Individuals with physical ill health.
- People who have experienced recent stressful events (e.g. divorce, bereavement).
- Those who make a definite statement with regard to plans involving a lethal method.
- Family history of suicide.
- History of deliberate self-harm.

- Prisoners.
- High-risk occupations (e.g. farmers, nurses, doctors).

Prevention

- Reduce risk in high-risk groups. Recognise if the patient belongs to a high-risk group, and specifically enquire about suicidal ideation. If the patient admits to suicidal thoughts, it is important that they are taken seriously and receive a full assessment. Improved community support facilities may be helpful.
- Ensure that healthcare professionals are adequately trained (two-thirds of people who commit suicide consult their GP in the month prior to their death).
- Reduce the availability and lethality of suicidal methods.
  - When the method of domestic gas production was changed in the 1960s, the content of carbon monoxide was reduced. This led to a marked decline in suicides due to domestic gas.
  - Since the availability of paracetamol and aspirin was reduced in 1998, deaths from poisoning have decreased by more than 20%.
- Improve public awareness.
- Reduce the stigma attached to mental illness.
- Promote research on suicide and suicide prevention.

Deliberate self-harm

This may be defined as intentionally self-inflicted harm without a fatal outcome. Deliberate self-harm is much more common than completed suicide, with an incidence of approximately 2 per 1000 population in the UK. It is much more frequent in women and in individuals under the age of 35 years. Common methods include self-poisoning and laceration. Precipitating factors include stressful life events (e.g. arguments with a boyfriend/girlfriend). Personality disorders are more common than psychiatric disorders among patients who deliberately self-harm, and alcohol abuse is often a problem.

Assessment of patients after deliberate self-harm

All patients should undergo a full assessment, as their risk of repeated self-harm is 20% in the next year and their risk of completed suicide is 1–2% in the following year (a 100-fold increase compared with the general population). It is important to obtain answers to the following questions.

- Was the act planned or carried out on impulse?
- Were precautions taken to avoid discovery?
- Did the patient seek help afterwards?
- Was the method dangerous?
- Was there a final act (e.g. making a will)?
- Does the patient express any regret?
- Do they now wish to die?
- What are the patient's current problems? Ask about their relationships with spouse/partner and children, financial issues, housing, employment and legal problems.
- Is there any evidence of psychiatric disorder?
- Is there a continuing risk of suicide or deliberate self-harm?

Only a small proportion of patients who deliberately self-harm will require admission for further management. The rest may be offered community-based follow-up.

Further reading

- Department of Health (2003) *National Suicide Prevention Strategy Launch: annual report.* Department of Health, London.
- Department of Health (1999) *Saving Lives: our healthier nation.* The Stationery Office, London.
- Barraclough BM, Bunch J, Nelson B and Sainsbury P (1974) A hundred cases of suicide: clinical aspects. *Br J Psychiatry.* **125**: 355–73.
- Department of Health (2002) *National Suicide Prevention Strategy for England.* The Stationery Office, London.
- Gelder M, Gath D, Mayou R and Cowen P (1996) *Oxford Textbook of Psychiatry* (3e). Oxford University Press, Oxford.

Delirium

Delirium (also known as acute confusional state) is a common condition, especially in hospital inpatients. Although it can be reversible in a significant proportion of cases, many patients will suffer further complications, have longer inpatient stays and also have a higher mortality rate.

Risk factors

- Elderly patients.
- Multiple medications.
- Post-operative patients.
- Pre-existing brain trauma.
- Alcohol dependence.
- Diabetes.
- Cancer.
- Sensory impairment.
- Malnutrition.

Diagnosis

- Altered level of consciousness – this is a characteristic feature. There is reduced ability to focus, sustain or shift attention.
- Global disturbance of cognition (e.g. memory registration, retention and recall) or development of perceptual disturbance.
- Disturbance develops over hours to days and fluctuates in severity.

Clinical features

- Fluctuations in severity (often worse at night).
- Behaviour may be marked by agitation or hypoactivity.
- Mood – patients may be apathetic, anxious, scared or perplexed. Affect is often labile.
- Disturbed thought processes may lead to incoherent speech.
- Perceptual abnormalities are common, and include illusions (misperceptions) and visual hallucinations.

- Delusions (often persecutory, and may be fleeting).
- Concentration is often impaired.
- Disorientation, particularly with regard to time.
- Disturbances of the sleep–wake cycle and activity are common.

Aetiology

Table 32   Aetiology of delirium

Drugs	Anticholinergic agents, anticonvulsants, anti-parkinsonism agents, steroids, cimetidine, opiates, benzodiazepines Alcohol and illicit drugs
Withdrawal syndromes	Alcohol, benzodiazepines, barbiturates
Systemic infections	Urinary tract infection, pneumonia, endocarditis, septicaemia Post-operative infection
Intracranial infections	Encephalitis, meningitis, brain abscess, HIV, cerebral malaria
Metabolic	Hypoxia Hypoglycaemia Disorders of electrolyte balance (Na^+ and Ca^{2+}) Disorders of fluid balance Endocrine disorders (e.g. hyper- or hypothyroidism) Rare causes (e.g. carcinoid syndrome, porphyria)
Cerebrovascular	Transient ischaemic attack, embolism, haemorrhage, migraine
Cardiovascular	Myocardial infarction, cardiac failure
Others	Head trauma Neoplastic disease Epilepsy Vitamin deficiency (e.g. thiamine, nicotinic acid) Pain, sleep deprivation and sensory deprivation

Management

Table 33   Management of delirium

Identify and treat the underlying cause	• This may be difficult as there are often multiple causes • Patients often cannot give a coherent history or co-operate with an examination • Information from carers and relatives may be useful
Environmental and supportive measures	• Clear communication (preferably from a single member of staff) • Orientation aids (e.g. clock faces, date written on whiteboard) • Correction of sensory impairments (e.g. by using spectacles and hearing aids) • Optimising environment (e.g. providing good lighting, reducing noise, removing dangerous objects) • Providing adequate warmth and nutrition
Medication for symptoms	• Drugs should only be used when essential (e.g. if patient is severely distressed or in danger of injuring him- or herself or others) • Antipsychotics are the first choice; elderly patients are at risk of side-effects, so low doses should be used (e.g. 500 mcg haloperidol) • Benzodiazepines may be used to treat withdrawal syndromes (e.g. delirium tremens), but care is necessary as they may exacerbate the underlying cause of the delirium (e.g. worsening hypoxia by causing respiratory depression) • A fixed dosing schedule is preferable to giving the drug 'as required'
Regular review	• An important area that is often neglected

Medico-legal issues

- There may be problems with regard to capacity and obtaining informed consent for treatments. A patient is deemed to have capacity if they can:
  - understand and retain information that is relevant to the decision in question
  - believe the information
  - weigh up the information in order to make an informed choice.

- Common law in the UK allows urgent interventions that are needed to prevent serious deterioration or death, so long as the doctor is acting in the best interests of the patient.

Further reading

- Gelder M *et al.* (eds) (2000*) New Oxford Textbook of Psychiatry.* Oxford University Press, Oxford.
- Brown TM and Boyle MF (2002) Delirium. In: R Mayou *et al.* (eds) *ABC of Psychological Medicine.* BMJ Books, London.

Alcohol withdrawal

Alcohol intoxication or withdrawal is one of the commonest presentations to Accident and Emergency departments in the UK. Simple management steps should always be taken to prevent serious complications of this condition.

Clinical features

- Tremor.
- Sweating.
- Tachycardia.
- Restlessness.
- Anxiety.
- Hypoglycaemia.
- Generalised seizure.

In the vast majority of cases, symptoms subside after 48 hours of cessation of alcohol. Delirium tremens is a severe form of alcohol withdrawal that develops around 3–4 days after cessation of alcohol. Although it only affects a minority of individuals, there is a high associated mortality rate. In addition to the other features of withdrawal, the patient may become pyrexial or develop psychotic features such as delusions or hallucinations.

Complications of alcohol abuse

- Aspiration pneumonia.
- Head injury, subdural haemorrhage.
- Liver failure.
- Wernicke's encephalopathy (nystagmus, 6th cranial nerve palsy, cerebellar ataxia and confusion).
- Korsakoff's syndrome (features of amnesia, psychosis and confabulation).
- Malnutrition.

Management

- Obtain IV access and give IV fluids to rehydrate the patient.
- Prescribe IV thiamine (Pabrinex, I + II) three times daily. This is a form of thiamine which prevents Wernicke–Korsakoff's syndrome (*see* above). *Note:* Pabrinex may rarely cause an anaphylactic

reaction, so should be given slowly over several minutes. Once the patient is able to take oral nutrition, they may be switched from Pabrinex to oral thiamine 100 mg twice daily.

● Multivitamins and B vitamins (compound strong) should also be prescribed.

● Chlordiazepoxide (Librium) is a long-acting benzodiazepine that reduces withdrawal symptoms by causing sedation. Prescribe a reducing dose such as that shown in Table 34.

Table 34 Suggested regimen for administration of chlordiazepoxide in cases of alcohol withdrawal

Day(s)	Oral chlordiazepoxide dose
1	15–20 mg six times daily
2	15 mg five times daily
3	10–15 mg four times daily
4	10 mg three times daily
5	10 mg twice daily
6–8	10 mg once daily

● If the patient continues to be agitated, try giving IV haloperidol (up to 10 mg).

● Check the blood sugar concentration, but only correct hypoglycaemia *after* Pabrinex has been given, in order to prevent precipitation of Wernicke's encephalopathy.

● If clotting is impaired, give vitamin K replacement.

Further reading

● American Society of Addiction Medicine, Committee on Practice Guidelines, Working Group on Pharmacological Management of Alcohol Withdrawal (1997) Pharmacological management of alcohol withdrawal: a meta-analysis and evidence-based practice guidelines. *JAMA.* **278:** 144–51.

17 Toxicology

Paracetamol overdose

Paracetamol is the drug most commonly taken in overdose in the UK, with an estimated 70 000 intentional overdoses occurring each year. In 2003, there were 87 deaths in England and Wales secondary to paracetamol overdose.

Aetiology

Paracetamol is primarily metabolised by the liver. After ingestion, the majority of the drug is conjugated and excreted. However, 5–10% is converted to the metabolite N-acetyl-p-benzoquinonimine (NAPQI), which is hepatotoxic and is normally inactivated by conjugation with glutathione. When large doses of paracetamol are ingested, hepatic glutathione is depleted and NAPQI binds directly to hepatocytes, causing cellular necrosis.

The recommended maximum daily dose of paracetamol is 4 g (or 8 tablets). Marked liver necrosis may be seen with an overdose of 10 g (20 tablets), and death with 15 g (30 tablets).

N-acetylcysteine may be used as an antidote to paracetamol, as it increases the availability of hepatic glutathione. It is most effective when infused within 8 hours of paracetamol ingestion, but it can provide protection for up to 24 hours after an overdose. Oral methionine is an alternative treatment if acetylcysteine cannot be administered promptly (e.g. in remote areas), but its absorption and efficacy are unreliable if the patient is vomiting.

Clinical features

- There are few symptoms in the first 24 hours after a paracetamol overdose, although some patients may complain of nausea and vomiting.
- The majority of patients recover within 48 hours.

- When liver failure occurs, it normally becomes apparent within 72–96 hours. Symptoms include jaundice, confusion and loss of consciousness.
- Acute renal failure may also occur (occasionally in the absence of significant liver damage).

Initial management

Treatment depends on the time of presentation after ingestion of a paracetamol overdose. The decision to give treatment is based on the plasma paracetamol concentration at least 4 hours after ingestion (as earlier samples may be misleading). The concentration is plotted on a paracetamol treatment graph (*see* Figure 16), and cases above the normal treatment line are treated with *N*-acetylcysteine.

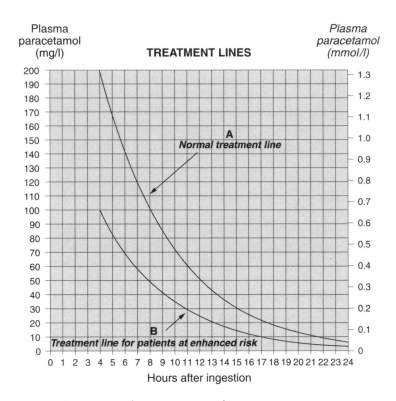

Figure 16   Paracetamol treatment graph

- Activated charcoal may help to prevent drug absorption if administered within 1 hour of ingestion. It should be considered in patients who have taken in excess of 150 mg/kg or 12 g of paracetamol (whichever is smaller).
- Gastric lavage is not recommended.
- Take blood samples as soon as possible when 4 hours or more have elapsed since the time of ingestion. Check U&Es, plasma glucose levels (hypoglycaemia may occur), LFTs, INR (the most sensitive marker of liver damage), blood pH and plasma paracetamol levels.
- Monitor fluid and electrolyte balance.
- Assess whether the patient is at increased risk of severe liver damage.
- Treat the patient if their plasma paracetamol concentration is above line A (or line B in high-risk groups) on the treatment graph.
- Treat the patient immediately with N-acetylcysteine if blood results will not be available within 8 hours of ingestion, or if the history suggests that there has been significant paracetamol ingestion *and* presentation is within 8–24 hours of the overdose.
- Plasma levels may be difficult to interpret if paracetamol has been taken over a number of hours. If there is any uncertainty, administer treatment.

High-risk groups

Patients in the following high-risk groups are more susceptible to liver damage and should be treated at lower concentrations of paracetamol:

- patients with glutathione deficiency (e.g. due to malnourishment, eating disorders or HIV)
- patients who are on enzyme-inducing drugs (e.g. carbamazepine, phenobarbital, phenytoin, primidone, rifampicin, St John's Wort)
- patients with a history of chronic excess alcohol intake.

N-acetylcysteine

- This is administered as an intravenous infusion diluted with 5% glucose as follows:
  - 150 mg/kg in 200 ml over 15 minutes
  - 50 mg/kg in 500 ml over 4 hours
  - 100 mg/kg in 1000 ml over 16 hours.
- It is important to monitor patients while treating them with N-acetylcysteine, as anaphylactoid reactions (urticarial rash, angio-oedema, bronchospasm or hypotension) occur in up to 15% of cases.

- If such reactions occur, stop the infusion and administer intravenous hydrocortisone and chlorpheniramine for severe reactions. Once the reaction has settled, restart the infusion at a lower rate.

Further management

- Repeat measurements of ALT, INR and serum creatinine levels once treatment is complete. The patient may be discharged if there are no abnormalities, but should be advised to return to hospital if vomiting or abdominal pain occurs.
- If any results are abnormal or the patient is symptomatic, further monitoring is required and advice must be sought from the National Poisons Information Service.
- A poor prognosis is indicated by an INR of > 3, raised serum creatinine levels or a blood pH of < 7.3 after 24 hours. If any of these findings are present, advice should be sought from a specialist liver unit.
- Since most paracetamol overdoses are deliberate, a psychiatric evaluation may be required prior to discharge.

Further reading

- Warrell D, Cox TM, Firth JD *et al.* (2003) *Oxford Textbook of Medicine* (4e). Oxford University Press, Oxford.
- Wallace CI, Dargan PI and Jones AL (2002) Paracetamol overdose: an evidence-based flowchart to guide management. *Emerg Med J.* **19**: 202–5.
- Paracetamol Information Centre; www.pharmweb.net/pwmirror/ pwy/paracetamol/pharmwebpic.html

Salicylate poisoning

Aetiology

Salicylate poisoning may result from a variety of sources, such as percutaneous absorption of salicylic acid (used in keratolytic agents) or ingestion of methyl salicylate (oil of wintergreen, a rubefacient), but is most commonly due to an oral overdose of aspirin.

- Salicylates are well absorbed from the stomach and small intestine. In overdose there may be delayed gastric emptying, so salicylate levels may continue to rise for up to 24 hours after ingestion (especially if enteric-coated tablets were ingested).
- Salicylate undergoes hepatic metabolism, a process that is saturated at therapeutic doses.
- Excess salicylate directly stimulates the respiratory centre, causing hyperventilation and a respiratory alkalosis.
- Compensatory mechanisms include the urinary excretion of bicarbonate together with potassium, sodium and water. This results in a metabolic acidosis.
- Salicylate also has effects on carbohydrate, lipid, protein and amino acid metabolism, which worsen the metabolic acidosis.
- Acidosis enhances the transfer of salicylate across the blood–brain barrier, thereby promoting its effects on the central nervous system (e.g. stupor).
- Children and the elderly are more susceptible to severe effects of salicylate, and at lower plasma levels.

Clinical features

Toxicity due to aspirin overdose may be crudely predicted on the basis of the dose ingested as shown in Table 35.

Table 35 Relationship between dose of aspirin ingested and estimated toxicity

Ingested dose (mg/kg body weight)	Estimated toxicity
< 150	Toxicity not expected
150–300	Mild to moderate toxicity
300–500	Severe toxicity
> 500	Potentially fatal

The symptoms that are observed will depend on the plasma levels of salicylate.

Table 36   Symptoms of salicylate toxicity

Mild (300–500 mg/litre)	Moderate (500–750 mg/litre)	Severe (> 750 mg/litre)
Burning of mouth	Tachypnoea	Hallucinations
Lethargy	Sweating	Stupor
Nausea	Dehydration	Convulsions
Vomiting	Hyperpyrexia	Pulmonary oedema
Dizziness	Loss of coordination	Renal failure
Tinnitus	Restlessness	Coma

Management

Early management

- Gastric lavage is recommended in adults only if in excess of 500 mg/kg aspirin was ingested less than 1 hour previously.
- Activated charcoal may be given to children and adults up to 12 hours after salicylate ingestion. Repeated doses may be required up to 4-hourly (particularly if enteric-coated tablets were ingested).

Intermediate management

- Check salicylate levels 2–4 hours after ingestion (as earlier levels may be difficult to interpret).
- Measure the levels again every 2–3 hours until the peak concentration is achieved and levels begin to fall.
- Monitor electrolytes, LFTs, serum glucose concentration and blood pH, as well as checking FBC and INR.
- Rehydrate the patient with oral/IV fluids, and correct any electrolyte imbalances.

Urinary alkalinisation (alkalisation)

- This enhances salicylate elimination and is indicated in patients with moderate or severe toxicity.
- Treat if the blood pH is < 7.3.
- In adults, administer 1 litre of 1.26% sodium bicarbonate with 20–40 mmol potassium as an IV infusion over 3 hours.

- In children, dilute 1 ml/kg 8.4% sodium bicarbonate and 1 mmol/kg potassium in 10 ml/kg sodium chloride solution and infuse at a rate of 2 ml/kg/hour.
- Check the urinary pH hourly and aim for a value in the range 7.5–8.5.
- Correct hypokalaemia (as this prevents urinary excretion of alkali). Aim for a serum potassium concentration of 4.0–4.5 mmol/l.
- Forced alkaline diuresis is not recommended due to the risk of fluid overload and pulmonary oedema.

Haemodialysis

- This is indicated in patients with severe toxicity or persistently raised salicylate concentrations that are unresponsive to urinary alkalinisation.
- Consider haemodialysis if the blood pH is < 7.2.

Discharge

- Once salicylate levels have fallen below 300 mg/litre in adults (or 200 mg/litre in children and the elderly) the patient can be discharged. However, they should be advised to return if they develop any symptoms such as vomiting, tinnitus or sweating.
- If the overdose was deliberate, organise a psychiatric evaluation prior to discharge.

Reye's syndrome

- This is a relatively rare condition characterised by acutely disturbed liver and brain function.
- Symptoms include vomiting, fever, altered consciousness, convulsions and coma.
- Salicylate therapy has been implicated as a causal agent, and aspirin is therefore contraindicated in children under the age of 12 years.

Further reading

- Warrell D, Cox TM, Firth JD *et al.* (2003) *Oxford Textbook of Medicine* (4e). Oxford University Press, Oxford.
- Dargan PI, Wallace CI and Jones AL (2002) An evidence-based flowchart to guide the management of acute salicylate (aspirin) overdose. *Emerg Med J.* **19**: 206–9.

Opiate overdose

Severe opiate intoxication tends to result from inadvertent overdose with illicit opiates such as heroin. However, it may also occur following overdose with compound analgesics. Opiates are responsible for the majority of deaths due to accidental self-poisoning.

Clinical features

Table 37   Clinical features of mild and severe opiate toxicity

Mild toxicity	Severe toxicity
Nausea	Respiratory depression
Vomiting	Pulmonary oedema
Drowsiness	Bradycardia
Constricted pupils	Clouded consciousness
Hypotension	Coma
Urticaria (with morphine and codeine)	

Note: These effects are potentiated by concomitant use of alcohol and psychotropic drugs.

Management

- Assess ABC.
- Establish a clear airway, adequate ventilation and oxygenation.
- Give oral activated charcoal, provided that the airway can be protected, if a substantial amount has been ingested within 2 hours.
- Naloxone is a competitive opiate antagonist and may be used as an antidote.
- Give intravenous naloxone (0.4 to 2 mg for an adult, and 0.01 mg/kg body weight for children) if coma or respiratory depression is present.
- Repeat the dose if there is no response within 2 minutes. Large doses (4 mg) may be required in cases of severe intoxication.
- Observe the patient carefully for recurrence of CNS effects or respiratory depression. Naloxone has a very short half-life so repeated doses may be required, especially if the overdose is due to a long-acting agent such as methadone.
- Intravenous infusions of naloxone may be useful if repeated doses are required.

- A particular concern is that the patient may abscond from hospital when they recover consciousness. This is particularly dangerous because naloxone is short-acting, so they may lapse into a coma and die unless further treatment is given. Intramuscular naloxone can be useful in these circumstances, as it may help to reduce the risk of respiratory arrest.

Further reading

- National Poisons Information Service (2002) *Opioid Analgesics: features and management.* National Poisons Information Service, London; www.spib.axl.co.uk/
- Warrell D, Cox TM, Firth JD *et al.* (2003) *Oxford Textbook of Medicine* (4e). Oxford University Press, Oxford.

Tricyclic antidepressant overdose

Tricyclic antidepressants are particularly dangerous drugs as they are often used in overdose, and are responsible for the vast majority of deaths from antidepressant overdose. In this class of drugs, dosulepin and amitriptyline appear to have the most toxic effects.

Aetiology

Tricyclic antidepressants have a number of toxic mechanisms, including the following:

- anticholinergic activity at autonomic nerve endings and in the brain
- sodium-channel blockade (effects on myocardium)
- inhibition of norepinephrine reuptake at nerve terminals
- vascular α-adrenergic blockade.

Clinical features

Anticholinergic effects

- Hot, dry skin.
- Dry mouth.
- Bowel ileus.
- Urinary retention.
- Confusion.

Cardiovascular effects

- Hypotension.
- Sinus tachycardia.
- Widened QRS duration (high risk of fits and arrhythmias).
- Ventricular arrhythmias (high risk of death).

Central nervous system effects

- Ataxia.
- Increased muscle tone, hyperreflexia and extensor plantar responses.
- Fixed and dilated pupils, divergent squint and nystagmus.
- Respiratory depression.
- Decreased level of consciousness.

- Rarely coma.
- Convulsions (> 5% cases).
- Agitation, delirium and visual hallucinations (especially during recovery).

Note: Patients may deteriorate rapidly (in less than 1 hour), so urgent hospital admission should be arranged for any patient in whom tricyclic antidepressant overdose is suspected.

Management

- Assess ABC – ensure that there is a clear airway and adequate ventilation.
- Establish intravenous access and take blood for U&Es. Correct any electrolyte abnormalities.
- Activated charcoal should be used if a large dose of tricyclic antidepressant has been taken in the last hour, so long as the airway can be protected. A second dose may be considered after 2 hours in patients with CNS symptoms who are able to swallow.
- Perform an ECG (looking in particular for prolonged QRS).
- Perform arterial blood gas analysis and correct hypoxia. If hypercapnia is present, assisted ventilation is indicated.
- Monitor urinary output.
- Cardiac monitoring should be undertaken. Observe the patient for 6 hours if they are asymptomatic. Patients who remain asymptomatic and have normal ECGs by 6 hours are unlikely to develop late complications.

Specific complications

Table 38   Specific complications of tricyclic antidepressant overdose

Arrhythmias	• These are best treated by correction of hypoxia and acidosis • Administer 50 mmol sodium bicarbonate to any patient with arrhythmias or significant ECG abnormalities (50 ml of 8.4% sodium bicarbonate, preferably through a central line due to its venous irritant effects). Repeated doses may be required • Do not administer anti-arrhythmic drugs, as they may worsen the arrhythmia
Hypotension	• Raise the foot of the bed • Expand the intravascular volume with intravenous fluids • Administer sodium bicarbonate as described above • Give glucagon 1 mg IV every 3 minutes if the patient is severely hypotensive; if there is a response to glucagon, consider starting an infusion at a rate of 2–4 mg/hour • Consider giving inotropes such as dopamine • Intra-aortic balloon pumping may be used in cases of extreme toxicity to correct hypotension
Convulsions	• Treat with IV diazepam (0.1–0.3 mg/kg body weight) or lorazepam (4 mg) • Phenytoin is contraindicated (as it blocks sodium channels and may increase the risk of cardiac arrhythmias) • If convulsions persist, consider intubation, paralysis, ventilation and further anticonvulsants
Delirium	• Treat with benzodiazepines; high doses (diazepam 20–30 mg every 2 hours) may be required • Avoid using major tranquillisers, as they may exacerbate hypotension and fits
Cardiac arrest	• Prolonged resuscitation (up to 1 hour) may be successful • Consider giving magnesium sulphate for refractory VF

Children

- Follow the same principles as described above, but contact the National Poisons Information Service for specialist advice.
- The use of sodium bicarbonate is controversial and should be guided by local policy and input from senior colleagues.
- Control convulsions with intravenous diazepam (from 0.2 mg/kg body weight up to a maximum of 0.6 mg/kg).
- Control delirium with oral diazepam. Treat children over 3 years of age with 0.4 mg/kg body weight. Children under 3 years are easier to control without sedation.
- Children are at increased risk of hypothermia.
- Treat any skin blisters as burns. Children should also be monitored for possible rhabdomyolysis.

Further reading

- National Poisons Information Service (1999) *Tricyclic Antidepressants: features and management.* National Poisons Information Service, London; www.spib.axl.co.uk/
- Ruben Thanacoody HK and Thomas SHL (2003) Antidepressant poisoning. *J R Coll Physicians Lond.* 3: 114–18.

18 Miscellaneous conditions

Shock

Shock is defined as a state in which tissue perfusion and oxygenation are inadequate to maintain organ function. This can be due to:

- respiratory failure, in which the tissues receive enough blood but the blood is not well oxygenated
- circulatory failure, which can be due to any of the following:
  - pump (cardiogenic) failure as a result of cardiac muscle failure, arrhythmias, valvular disease, obstruction due to pulmonary embolus, or coronary heart disease
  - a lack of circulating volume (hypovolaemia) due to blood loss, fluid loss (e.g. in burns patients), intestinal obstruction or peritonitis
  - fluid maldistribution due to sepsis or anaphylaxis.

The impaired tissue perfusion and resultant ischaemia result in the formation of lactic acid and a consequent metabolic acidosis, which is best assessed by measuring arterial blood gases. If left untreated, shock can lead to multiple organ dysfunction syndrome or failure, which has a high mortality.

Diagnosis

The clinical features of shock can be determined from the relevant cardiac physiology:

cardiac output = stroke volume × heart rate

blood pressure = cardiac output × peripheral vascular resistance.

The tissues are receiving poorly oxygenated blood, so the body tries to compensate by increasing cardiac output. This is achieved by increasing the heart rate. *Thus an early sign of shock is tachycardia.* The body also tries to maintain the blood pressure so that oxygen can reach the tissues. Therefore the sympathetic nervous system is activated to produce peripheral vasoconstriction and increase the peripheral vascular resistance, thus maintaining the blood pressure until the latter stages of shock. This vasoconstriction leads to cold, clammy peripheries, and the patient appears dehydrated ('peripheral shutdown').

The body also tries to compensate by increasing oxygenation. Therefore the respiratory rate increases. The kidneys cease to produce urine in an attempt to maintain the circulating volume, but this is a late sign. The lack of blood flow to the brain with increasing shock causes confusion and drowsiness as late signs.

Different types of shock may have slightly different features. For example, in neurogenic shock the sympathetic failure means that there is no tachycardia, and in septic shock the peripheries are warm due to the inflammatory response.

Management

Maintenance of oxygen delivery is the key to improving survival. Early aggressive management is often the only way to prevent mortality, and it is imperative that specialist medical advice is sought for any patient suspected of being in shock.

The aim of treatment is resuscitation (ABC) (*see* p. 149). This allows maximisation of oxygen delivery to the tissues. 'A' and 'B' are maintained with adequate ventilatory support and oxygenation. 'C', which is compromised in haemorrhagic shock, is managed by controlling any obvious sources of bleeding with direct pressure and elevation, fluid replacement and cardiac support (*see* p. 156).

Cardiac support to improve pump function may also be required, as the blood not only needs to be well oxygenated but must also be pumped to the tissues. This is achieved by maintaining a good cardiac output by increasing stroke volume (using inotropes) or heart rate (using chronotropes). In order to monitor the response to cardiac drugs and fluid resuscitation, the patient may have a CVP line inserted, typically into one of the internal jugular or subclavian veins. This allows monitoring of the pressure inside the right atrium of the heart, which provides an indirect measure of left ventricular pressure and therefore the volume status of the patient. Further fluid resuscitation and cardiac support can then be tailored to the CVP and clinical state of the patient. However, certain conditions make the CVP an unreliable indicator of volume status (e.g.

myocardial infarction, tension pneumothorax, air embolism, cardiac contusion, pericardial effusion).

Monitoring

Regular monitoring is essential during shock, so that treatment can be constantly titrated to response. The heart rate, blood pressure, respiratory rate, urinary output, temperature, conscious level, CVP, blood tests and ABG should be regularly assessed. Once the patient is stabilised, they may need to be transferred to a higher level of care where such monitoring is readily available.

Further reading

- Dobb GJ (2002) Circulatory shock. In: TE Oh (ed.) *Intensive Care Manual* (4e). Butterworth-Heinemann, Edinburgh.
- Archbold A (2001) Clinical assessment and invasive monitoring of volume status, cardiac output, and systemic vascular resistance. In: R Ashford and N Evans (eds) *Surgical Critical Care*. Greenwich Medical Media Ltd, London.
- Colvin JR (2000) Hypotension (Critical Care: Module 2). In: IMA Ledingham (ed.) *RCSE SELECT Programme*. Centre for Medical Education, University of Dundee, Dundee.

Sepsis and its sequelae

Definitions

- Systemic inflammatory response syndrome (SIRS) is a harmful excessive reaction of the acute-phase response defined by any two of the following:
  - temperature > 38°C or < 36°C
  - tachycardia > 90 beats/minute
  - tachypnoea >20 breaths/minute
  - white blood count > 12×10^9 or < 4×10^9.
- Sepsis is the development of SIRS due to infection.
- Severe sepsis is defined as sepsis plus organ dysfunction.
- Septic shock is defined as severe sepsis plus hypotension (despite fluid resuscitation).
- Septicaemia refers to the clinical signs and symptoms associated with the presence of pathogens in the bloodstream.
- Bacteraemia is defined as the presence of bacteria in the bloodstream, and is not necessarily symptomatic nor does it always require treatment.

Pathology

The inflammatory response is mediated by cytokines and growth factors such as interleukins, tumour necrosis factor and transforming growth factor beta. It is important to remember that immunocompromised patients (e.g. those with HIV/AIDS, diabetes, transplant or malnutrition) can be septic without eliciting a significant inflammatory response.

Pathogens vary depending on the site of the infection, but typically include the following:

- skin – Gram-positive cocci
- wound – Gram-positive cocci, enterococci, *E. coli*, *Pseudomonas*
- gastrointestinal/urological – Gram-negative, *E. coli*, *Enterobacter*, *Proteus*, methicillin-resistant *Staphylococcus aureus* (MRSA).

Clinical features

With the onset of SIRS, vasodilatation of vessels mediated by nitric oxide (also known as endothelium-derived relaxing factor) occurs. The clinical effects include the following:

- flushed, warm peripheries (this differentiates septic shock from other shock states)
- hypotension
- tachycardia
- hypoxia
- metabolic acidosis on ABG analysis (due to hypoperfusion and lactic acid accumulation as a result of hypoxia)
- impaired clotting (as the clotting cascade is affected by the inflammatory response).

Overt signs of inflammation may be seen at the site of infection in many cases of sepsis. There are four cardinal signs of inflammation:

1 dolor (pain)
2 calor (heat)
3 rubor (redness or erythema)
4 tumor (swelling).

Investigations

Routine blood parameters of inflammation such as white blood count and C-reactive protein will be raised. The site of sepsis should be sought by examining surgical sites and wounds, cannula sites, urine microscopy, culture and sensitivities (especially if the patient is catheterised), chest examination, chest X-ray and sputum culture, and ultrasound examination for potential fluid accumulation. It is often necessary to change catheters, IV and arterial lines, and to send their tips off for culture, as well as performing repeated blood cultures (using an aseptic technique and undertaking this before commencing antibiotic therapy).

Management

This will vary depending on the severity of the condition and the precipitating cause, but the basic principles are as follows.

- Evaluate ABC first (this includes the administration of high-flow oxygen).

- Give fluid resuscitation in order to restore organ perfusion and oxygenation (a urinary catheter plus a CVP or Swann–Ganz catheter should be considered in order to monitor fluid status accurately).
- Acid–base status should be monitored regularly by measuring ABG.
- In severe cases, haemodynamic support to maintain intravascular volume may be required. Noradrenaline (norepinephrine) will increase peripheral vascular resistance and achieve this (these patients are ill enough to warrant ITU management).
- Treat empirically with broad-spectrum antibiotics, employing a 'best-guess' approach until definitive antimicrobial therapy can be instituted based on sensitivity results (and often also advice from the microbiology department).
- Identify the precipitating cause and treat it with antibiotics and drainage if an abscess is found.
- If the condition does not resolve rapidly, consider giving the patient nutritional support (preferably enteral, unless the gastrointestinal tract is involved, in which case total parenteral nutrition should be used).

Multi-organ dysfunction syndrome (MODS)/multi-organ failure (MOF)

If SIRS is not treated adequately and promptly, it can progress to multi-organ dysfunction syndrome (MODS). This is defined as reversible dysfunction of two or more organs as a result of the hypoperfusion and consequent ischaemia that result from a continuing inflammatory process. The clinical features will depend on the organs affected, and can be summarised as follows:

- respiratory – hypoxia, respiratory failure, acute respiratory distress syndrome
- cardiovascular – oedema due to fluid extravasation out of the vessels into the tissues, hypotension resulting from a decrease in peripheral vascular resistance (due to nitric oxide-mediated vasodilatation), lactic acidosis due to the resulting hypoxia, myocardial ischaemia/infarction resulting from the above together with the direct effects of inflammatory mediators and endotoxins released
- renal – oliguria due to reduced renal perfusion and filtration
- hepatic – reduced clearance of metabolites and drugs, jaundice, abnormal clotting and DIC, reduced immunity
- gastrointestinal tract – atrophy of villi causes bacterial translocation which aggravates the SIRS and thus exacerbates the MODS

- cerebral – brain ischaemia is manifested as confusion, sedation or agitation
- haematological – bleeding caused by DIC.

If MODS continues, the organs become irreversibly damaged and multi-organ failure (MOF) results. However, effective management of MODS should prevent this.

Management

Aim to:

1 support the affected organs
2 improve tissue perfusion and oxygenation.

Organs are supported by a variety of complex ITU techniques (e.g. ventilation, inotropic support, dialysis), and this is best done by experienced intensive-care specialists. However, the delivery of oxygen can be maximised by anyone who remembers that it is proportional to cardiac output, haemoglobin levels and oxygen saturation.

We also know that cardiac output = stroke volume × heart rate, and that cardiac output = blood pressure/peripheral vascular resistance. Therefore the delivery of oxygen to the tissues can be optimised by:

- increasing stroke volume by giving chronotropic support
- increasing heart rate by giving inotropic support
- increasing blood pressure by using α-agonists
- increasing haemoglobin levels using transfusion as necessary
- increasing oxygen saturation using high-flow oxygen or mechanical ventilation.

Prognosis

The prognosis for patients with MODS/MOF depends on age, comorbidity, extent of sepsis and (crucially) the number of organs that have failed and how long they remain failed. With two failed organs the mortality rate after 24 hours is 50%, and after 72 hours it is 65%. With three failed organs these figures rise to 80% and 95%, respectively.

Further reading

- Brealey D and Singer M (2000) Multi-organ dysfunction in the critically ill: effects on different organs. *J R Coll Physicians Lond.* 34: 428–31.

- Brealey D and Singer M (2000) Multi-organ dysfunction in the critically ill: epidemiology, pathophysiology and management. *J R Coll Physicians Lond.* **34**: 124–7.
- Baue AE (1999) Sepsis, multi-organ dysfunction syndrome (MODS) and multiple organ failure (MOF). Prevention is better than treatment. *Minerva Anestesiol.* **65**: 477 81.

Anaphylaxis

Anaphylaxis is an acute, severe and systemic type I hypersensitivity reaction. Rapid treatment is vital, as this condition may cause life-threatening airways obstruction and shock.

Causes of anaphylaxis

Any allergy may cause anaphylaxis if it is severe enough. Common allergies include the following:

- drugs:
  - β-lactam antibiotics (e.g. penicillins, cephalosporins)
  - aspirin
- food products (e.g. peanuts)
- pollen
- house dust mite
- animals (e.g. cats).

Clinical features

- Skin manifestations such as erythema and urticaria (acute swelling in the skin).
- Irritation of mucous membranes, causing conjunctivitis and rhinitis.
- Stridor, indicating laryngeal oedema and obstruction.
- Bronchospasm (with expiratory wheeze), causing obstruction of lower airways.
- Cardiovascular complications such as hypotension and shock.

Management

- Commence high-flow oxygen via a mask.
- Treat any bronchospasm as for an acute asthma attack with repeated salbutamol nebulisers 2.5–5 mg.
- If the patient develops stridor and their breathing becomes laboured, an anaesthetist should be called immediately to perform emergency intubation. Alternatively, a cricothyroidotomy should be performed by insertion of a 14G cannula into the cricothyroid membrane of the larynx.
- *Intramuscular* adrenaline (epinephrine) 0.5–1 mg (1 in 1000 dilution) should be administered without delay.

- Check the patient's blood pressure. If they are hypotensive, 1–2 litres of IV fluids should be given rapidly.
- If life-threatening shock is present, consider slow *intravenous* injection of adrenaline 0.5–1 mg (1 in 10 000 dilution; *note the different concentration to adrenaline used intramuscularly*). However, this should only be done by an experienced healthcare professional.
- Give IV chlorpheniramine 10–20 mg (an antihistamine).
- Give IV hydrocortisone 100–500 mg for severe or recurrent reactions, or in the presence of asthma.
- Stop any drug or other agent suspected of precipitating the attack.

Further reading

- Resuscitation Council (UK) (2002) *The Emergency Medical Treatment of Anaphylactic Reactions for First Medical Responders and for Community Nurses.* Resuscitation Council (UK), London.

Post-operative pyrexia

There are many causes of a fever after surgery. Surgery itself stimulates an acute inflammatory response, with the release of pyrogenic cytokines such as interleukin-1. Thus pyrexia within the first 24 post-operative hours is often normal. However, continued pyrexia, especially of a swinging nature, is an indication of infection. The differential diagnosis includes the following:

- wound infection
- cannula site infection
- chest infection
- thromboembolism (see p. 81)
- urinary tract infection
- enterocolitis
- drug reaction (see p. 258)
- deep-seated abscess (e.g. pelvic abscess after abdominal or pelvic surgery).

Careful examination of the wound and cannula sites, chest, calves and abdomen, together with inspection of the drug chart, and simple investigations such as X-rays, urine dipstick and stool culture will help to determine the exact cause.

Wound infection

Any operation can become infected, since epithelia are broken and/or foreign instrumentation is introduced. In cases associated with pre-operative sepsis, post-operative infection rates are high. Meticulous attention to sterile technique and tissue handling is imperative in order to prevent infections if at all possible. All sites of potential infection should be carefully debrided and dressed appropriately. The organisms most commonly involved in post-operative infection are *Staphylococcus aureus* (including MRSA), *Streptococcus faecalis*, *Pseudomonas*, coliforms and *Bacteroides*.

Typically, wound (surgical site) infections occur around day 5 after the operation, but may present later if antibiotics have been used. The following characteristic signs of inflammation are present at the wound site:

- dolor (pain)
- calor (heat)

- rubor (redness)
- tumor (swelling).

The patient may also exhibit systemic features of infection, including the following:

- malaise
- anorexia
- vomiting
- swinging pyrexia.

Established infection is treated by giving antibiotics if it is cellulitis, and by drainage if there is pus. Release of sutures or surgical clips may allow pus to escape and aid resolution of the infection.

Cannula site infection

Any cannula associated with signs of inflammation should be removed and another one inserted at another site. Skin organisms, such as *Staphylococcus* and *Streptococcus*, are the commonest cause, and can be managed with a 5-day oral course of flucloxacillin. Because infection is almost inevitable in any cannula that is left *in situ* for more than 5 days, *all* cannulae should be changed every 3–5 days.

Chest infection

Almost all abdominal and thoracic operations will result in some degree of lung collapse within the first few post-operative hours. This is due to the increased mucus retention that results from surgery. The mucus retention causes blockage of distal bronchioles, resulting in the collapse of the supplied lung segments. The collapsed lung segments (usually basal, due to the effects of gravity and the ventilation/perfusion gradients in different regions of the lungs) may become secondarily infected with inhaled or aspirated organisms, leading to chest infection (typically around 1 week post-operatively). Rarely, lung abscess may result. Typical signs of chest infection include dyspnoea, tachycardia, pyrexia, cyanosis and difficulty in coughing. Physiotherapy may aid the expectoration of sputum. Purulent sputum is a clear sign of chest infection, and warrants culture and antibiotic treatment based on sensitivity results. In the interim, empirical treatment to cover hospital-acquired pneumonia (e.g. co-amoxyclav or a third-generation cephalosporin) should be instituted to cover *Streptococcus pneumoniae*, *Pseudomonas* and other common organisms.

Urinary tract infection

Urinary tract infection (UTI) is a broad term used to describe an inflammatory response of urothelium to an infectious agent. UTIs can involve either the upper urinary tract (kidneys) or the lower urinary tract (bladder and urethra). Most of these infections are caused by bacteria (*E. coli* accounts for 80–90% of cases). Urinalysis will show bacteriuria with pyuria (bacterial organisms and leukocytes in the urine). Most uncomplicated UTIs respond well to a 3- to 5-day course of oral antimicrobial agents. Trimethoprim is often used, but in many geographical areas UTIs are resistant to this drug, and first-line therapy then consists of a quinolone such as ciprofloxacin. If symptoms persist, it is important to take a urine culture and adjust treatment on the basis of the sensitivity results.

In cases of severe acute pyelonephritis, many patients require hospital admission for treatment with IV antimicrobial agents and hydration. In pregnancy, even asymptomatic bacteriuria should be treated, as the anatomical and physiological changes associated with pregnancy increase the risk of pyelonephritis, which can in turn lead to premature delivery and other complications.

Enterocolitis

Broad-spectrum antibiotics such as cephalosporins (e.g. cefotaxime) and clindamycin destroy the normal commensal gut flora and allow the development of resistant strains, such as the toxin-producing *Clostridium difficile* (formerly *welchii*). The toxins cause mucosal inflammation and pseudomembrane formation (pseudomembranous colitis), resulting in watery diarrhoea. This typically presents within the first week after antibiotic use, with loss of fluid and resultant shock, and sometimes with toxic dilatation of the colon.

Management is supportive and consists of giving IV fluid and electrolyte replacement, withdrawing the offending antibiotic, starting metronidazole or vancomycin, and keeping the patient nil by mouth until an improvement is seen.

Abscess

Deep-seated abscess typically presents with a swinging pyrexia for 2–3 weeks post-operatively. Investigations such as X-ray, ultrasound examination and CT scanning are usually diagnostic. Management is by drainage, either radiologically or surgically. *Antibiotics do not treat pus, drainage does.*

Further reading

- Smith RC and Ledingham IMA (2000) Pyrexia (Critical Care: Module 13). In: *The RCSE SELECT Programme.* Centre for Medical Education, University of Dundee, Dundee.
- Smith JAR (1999) Complications – prevention and management. In: RM Kirk, AO Mansfield and JPS Cochrane (eds) *Clinical Surgery in General* (3e). Churchill Livingstone, London.
- Cunningham R and Dance D (2001) Infection in surgery. In: A Kingsnorth and A Majid (eds) *Principles of Surgical Practice.* Greenwich Medical Media Ltd, London.

Acute pain management

Different analgesics work by interfering with different parts of the pain pathway. For example, local anaesthetics work by blocking nerve action potentials, NSAIDs such as aspirin work by inhibiting the production of certain inflammatory mediators (prostaglandins and leukotrienes), opiates such as morphine inhibit the spinal cord dorsal horn (by acting on μ-receptors) and thereby prevent the transmission of pain, and α-2-adrenergic agonists such as tizanidine and clonidine exert their effect by reducing the central transmission of painful stimuli.

Paracetamol

Paracetamol (acetaminophen) is a peripherally acting drug with no anti-inflammatory activity. It has approximately the same analgesic activity as aspirin, and is a useful analgesic and anti-pyretic (it reduces fever). Paracetamol does not cause gastric irritation and is remarkably safe. However, in overdose it can cause liver damage. Up to 4 g daily is the maximum dose for an adult, but paracetamol toxicity is increased by alcohol, barbiturates and possibly zidovudine.

Non-steroidal anti-inflammatory drugs (NSAIDs)

NSAIDs are the mainstay of treatment of mild and moderate pain associated with tissue inflammation. Due to their ability to block the enzyme cyclo-oxygenase (COX), NSAIDs have analgesic, anti-inflammatory and antipyretic actions. It is the inhibition of COX-2 that accounts for the beneficial effects of NSAIDs. COX-1 inhibition is responsible for their adverse side-effects (e.g. gastric ulceration, renal failure and increasing bleeding tendency). Therefore NSAIDs should not be used in patients with renal impairment, bleeding tendency or a history of peptic ulcer disease.

Newer drugs that are COX-2-specific inhibitors have recently become available (e.g. celecoxib, rofecoxib), which offer the promise of the beneficial analgesic effects without the unwanted side-effects. However, their side-effect profile has yet to be fully determined, and initial suspicions of long-term cardiac toxicity have led to the withdrawal of rofecoxib from the market and strict warnings about the use of other COX-2-specific drugs. At the time of writing, the advice from the Department of Health is that these drugs should only be prescribed for patients with no significant cardiovascular morbidity or risk factors, and that they should be used at the lowest possible dosage for the shortest possible time.

Opiates

Opiates exert analgesic actions primarily by blocking μ receptors, and are mostly morphine derivatives. Although opiates have profound analgesic effects, they also have potentially lethal side-effects, including the following:

- respiratory depression
- bradycardia
- altered conscious state (confusion, sedation or euphoria), which is particularly marked in the elderly
- constipation
- pupillary constriction (pinpoint pupils are often a sign of opiate overdose)
- nausea and vomiting (therefore an anti-emetic should always be given when administering opiates).

Any patient with suspected opiate-induced respiratory depression that reduces their oxygen saturations (measured with a pulse oximeter) should be given an opiate antagonist such as naloxone to reverse the effect. As the duration of action of naloxone is shorter than that of most opiates, it should be given as an initial intravenous bolus (typically 400 μg) and then as a continuous infusion.

Opiates have traditionally been given by mouth (e.g. Oramorph) or by intermittent IM injection for post-operative pain relief (e.g. 10 mg up to every 4 hours as needed). This inevitably leads to peaks and troughs in the blood concentrations of the drug, with resultant peaks and troughs in both pain relief and side-effects. Continuous repeated small intravenous boluses (e.g. 1 mg up to every 5 minutes as needed) are therefore becoming more usual, as is the case with patient-controlled analgesia (PCA). PCA also allows patients to control their own analgesia, which in itself results in a decreased analgesic requirement. Opiates (e.g. diamorphine and fentanyl) may also be given by anaesthetists via an epidural route, often in combination with local anaesthetics. This regime is commonly used for post-operative patients.

Analgesic ladder

The analgesic ladder is summarised in Figure 17.

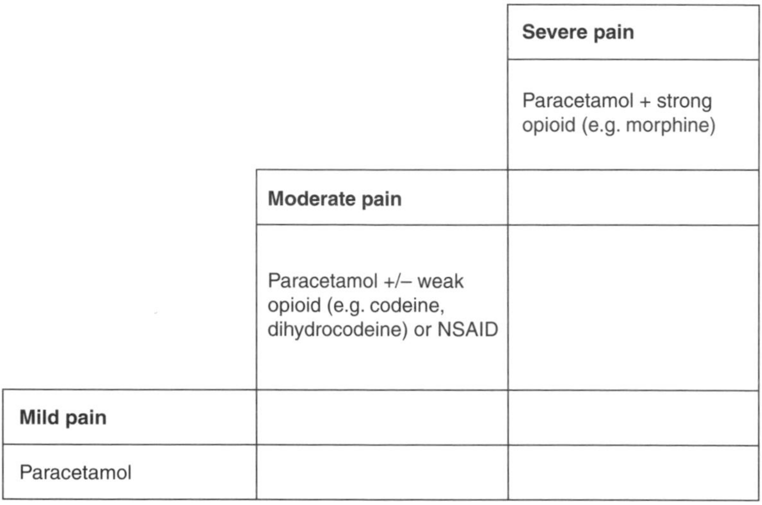

		Severe pain
		Paracetamol + strong opioid (e.g. morphine)
	Moderate pain	
	Paracetamol +/– weak opioid (e.g. codeine, dihydrocodeine) or NSAID	
Mild pain		
Paracetamol		

Figure 17   Analgesic ladder

If uncontrollable pain is experienced with the above regime, this should prompt referral to an anaesthetist for the use of specialist agents (e.g. clonidine, ketamine) or techniques (e.g. local anaesthetic regional blocks).

Further reading

- Skinner HB (2004) Multimodal acute pain management. *Am J Orthop*. **33 (Suppl. 5)**: 5–9.
- Burris JE (2004) Pharmacologic approaches to geriatric pain management. *Arch Phys Med Rehabil*. **85 (Suppl. 3)**: S45–9.
- Fernando R and Hunt KD (1999) The management of postoperative pain. In: RM Kirk, AO Mansfield and JPS Cochrane (eds) *Clinical Surgery in General* (3e). Churchill Livingstone, London.

Index

ABC evaluation 1–3, 149–50, 251
abdominal aortic aneurysms,
    rupture 134–5
ABO incompatibility 95
abscess 262–3
acute asthma 31–4
acute confusional states 231–4
acute coronary syndrome (ACS)
    13–16
acute glaucoma 177–8
acute limb ischaemia 139–40
acute pancreatitis 102–5
acute peritonitis 107–9
acute psychosis 221–7
acute pulmonary oedema 25–6
acute pyelonephritis 132, 262
acute renal failure (ARF) 59–61
acute transfusion reaction 94–6
acute urine retention 130–1
Addisonian crisis 78–80
adrenal glands
    cortical insufficiency 78–80
    medullary tumours 76–7
advanced life support
    adults 149, 152–7
    paediatrics 199
    see also cardiopulmonary
        resuscitation
age-related macular
    degeneration 181
airways obstruction 2
    facial injuries 183
    management principles 152–3
alcohol withdrawal 235–6
allergic reactions, anaphylaxis
    258–9
AMD (age-related macular
    degeneration) 181
amitriptyline overdose 246–9
AMPLE history 150–6

analgesic ladder 266
anaphylaxis 258–9
angiodysplasia 124
aortic dissection 136–8
aplastic crisis 92
appendicitis 99–101
ARF (acute renal failure) 59–61
ascending cholangitis 106
aspirin overdose 241–3
asthma 31–4
    life-threatening exacerbation
        33–4
asystole
    adults 11–12
    paediatrics 199
ATLS (Advanced Trauma Life
    Support) system 149
ATOMFC mnemonic 150
atrial fibrillation 18–19
atrial flutter 17
AVPU mnemonic 150

bacteraemia 253
bacterial meningitis 48–50
basic life support (BLS) 1–4
    cardiopulmonary resuscitation
        3
    paediatric 198
battered baby syndrome 194–6
Beck's triad 29–30
benign prostatic hypertrophy
    (BPH) 130
bile duct infections 106
bladder stones 128–9
blood products, transfusion
    reactions 94–6
'blue bloaters' 35–8
bowel obstructions
    large 114–16
    small 117

BPH (benign prostatic
    hypertrophy)   130
bradycardia   22–4
brainstem, coning   49, 158
breathing problems   2, 31–42
    asthma   31–4
    COPD   35–8
    pneumothorax   39–41, 154–5
    management principles   154–5
broad complex tachycardia   20–1
Brown–Sequard syndrome   143
Brudzinski's sign   49
burn injuries   165–8
    non-accidental paediatric   195

caecal rupture   115–16
cannula site infections   261
cardiac arrest
    asystole   11–12, 199
    chest compressions   2–3, 198
    diagnosis   2
    and drowning   162
    and hypothermia   164
    paediatric   197–9
    pulseless electrical activity   8–10
    ventricular fibrillation   5–7
cardiac tamponade   9, 29–30
cardiopulmonary resuscitation
    (CPR)   3, 5–6, 149–50, 251
carotid pulse   2
carotid sinus massage   17
cauda equina syndrome   131, 145
central retinal artery occlusion   179
central retinal vein occlusion
    179–80
cerebral haemorrhage   54–5
    cf. stroke   51–3
cerebrospinal fluid
    analysis   50
    otorrhoea/rhinorrhoea   159
cerebrovascular accident   51–3
Charcot's triad   106
chest compressions
    adults   2–3
    paediatrics   198
child abuse   194–6
cholangitis   106

chronic bronchitis, exacerbation
    35–6
chronic obstructive pulmonary
    disease (COPD)   35–8
circulation trauma, management
    principles   156–7
CO_2 retention   36–8
coma   43–5
compartment syndrome   146–7
confusional states   231–4
coning   49, 158
conjunctivitis   177
consent issues   233–4
convulsions   248
COPD (chronic obstructive
    pulmonary disease)   35–8
cord prolapse   211–12
corneal disease   177
CPR (cardiopulmonary
    resuscitation)   3, 5–6,
    149–50, 251
croup   188
CSF (cerebrospinal fluid)
    analysis   50
CT scans, head injuries   159
Cullen's sign   103
Cushing's reflex   46

de-escalation techniques   225–6
deep vein thrombosis (DVT)   81–2
defibrillation   5–6
deliberate self-harm   229–30
delirium   231–4
diabetic ketoacidosis (DKA)   66–9
DIC (disseminated intravascular
    coagulopathy)   86–7
disseminated intravascular
    coagulopathy (DIC)   86–7
    and placental abruption   207
diverticular disease   124–5
DKA (diabetic ketoacidosis)   66–9
dosulepin overdose   246–9
drowning   161–2
duodenal ulceration   121–3

eclampsia   210
ectopic pregnancy   201–3

electrolyte levels, potassium
    disturbances 62–3
electromechanical dissociation *see*
    pulseless electrical activity
    (PEA)
embolisms
    acute limb ischaemia 139–40
    pulmonary 83–5
emphysema, exacerbation 35–6
enterocolitis 262
epiglottitis 188–9
epileptic seizures 56–8
epistaxis 185–6
erythema multiforme major
    173
erythroderma 171–2
eye conditions
    acute glaucoma 177–8
    conjunctivitis 177
    corneal disease 177
    haemorrhage 176–7
    iridocyclitis 177
    optic neuritis 178
    see also vision loss

facial injuries 182–4
febrile convulsions 190–2
fetus, shoulder dystocia 213–14
flail chest 155
fluid replacement regimes 156–7
    burn injuries 166–8
    paediatrics 200
    pre-eclampsia 209
fractures 141–2, 169
    paediatric non-accidental 195

gastric ulceration 121–3
gastrointestinal bleeding
    lower tract 124–5
    upper tract 121–3
Glasgow Coma Scale 43, 158
glaucoma, acute 177–8
gout, acute 148
Grey–Turner's sign 103

haemarthrosis 148
haemodialysis 61

haemorrhage, management
    principles 156–7
haemorrhoids 125
HATI (human anti-tetanus
    immunoglobulin) 170
head injuries 158–60
heart block 22–4
HELLP syndrome 209
hepatic encephalopathy 110–12
hernias, strangulated 117,
    119–20
heroin overdose 244–5
history taking, trauma 150–6
hyper-osmolar non-ketotic acidosis
    (HONK) 70–3
hyperkalaemia 9, 61, 62–3
hypersensitivity reactions 258–9
hypertension
    malignant (accelerated) 27–8
    and pre-eclampsia 208–10
hypoglycaemia 74–5
hypokalaemia 9
hypothermia 9, 162–4
hypovolaemia 8

ICP (intracranial pressure) 46–7,
    158–60
informed consent, patient
    capacity 233–4
intracerebral haemorrhage 54–5
iridocyclitis 177
ischaemia
    limb 139–40
    optic neuropathy 180

joints, acute inflammation 148

keratitis 177
Kernig's sign 49
Kussmaul's sign 29–30, 66

large bowel obstruction
    114–16
life support measures
    adult 1–4, 5–6, 149–50, 251
    paediatric 198–9
limb ischaemia 139–40

liver failure 110–13
  paracetamol overdose 237–40
  transplantation criteria 113
lower gastrointestinal bleeding
    124–5
lumbar punctures 50
  contraindications 47

McRoberts' position 213
macular degeneration 181
malignant hypertension 27–8
Mallory–Weiss tear 121–3
MANTREL score 99–100
massive haemothorax 155
maxillofacial trauma 182–4
medico-legal issues, delirium 233–4
meningitis 48–50
Mental Health Act (1983) 227
mental state examination 223
mesenteric infarction 118
mesenteric ischaemia 118
microangiopathic haemolytic
    anaemia (MAHA) 86–7
MODS (multi-organ dysfunction
    syndrome) 106, 255–7
Mount Vernon formula 167–8
MRSA, and sepsis 253
multi-organ failure/dysfunction
    (MOF/DS) 106, 255–7
myocardial ischaemia
  full-thickness (Q wave) 14,
      15–16
  non-ST-elevation 14

N-acetylcysteine 237, 239–40
narrow complex tachycardia 179
neuroglycopenia 74–5
neurological examination 45
  Glasgow Coma Scale 43, 158
neuropraxia 143
neutropenic sepsis 88–90
nose bleeds 185–6
NSAIDs (non-steroidal anti-
    inflammatory drugs) 264–6

oesophageal varices 122–3
open pneumothorax 154–5

opiates
  overdose 244–5
  pain management 265–6
optic neuritis 178

paediatrics 187–200
  cardiorespiratory arrest 197–9
  croup 188
  epiglottitis 188–9
  febrile convulsions 190–2
  non-accidental injury 194–6
  pyloric stenosis 192–3
  stridor 187–9
  trauma 199–200
pain management 264–6
pancreatitis, acute 102–5
paracetamol
  overdose 237–40
  pain management 264, 266
patient capacity 233–4
PEA (pulseless electrical activity)
    8–10
  and cardiac tamponade 29–30
pericardiocentesis 30
peritonitis, acute 107–9
phaeochromocytoma 76–7
'pink puffers' 35–8
placenta praevia 204–5
placental abruption 206–7
pneumothorax 39–41, 154–5
  primary 39, 41
  secondary 39, 42
portal hypertension 111–12
post-operative pyrexia 260–3
postpartum haemorrhage 215–17
potassium disturbances
  hyperkalaemia 62–3
  rhabdomyolysis 64–5
praecordial thump 5
pre-eclampsia 208–10
pre-renal failure 60
priapism 133
proteinuria, in pre-eclampsia
    208–10
psychosis, acute presentation 221–7
pulmonary embolism (PE) 83–5
pulmonary oedema 25–6, 60–1

pulseless electrical activity (PEA)
    8–10
    and cardiac tamponade   29–30
pulsus paradoxus   29–30
pus   263
pyelonephritis, acute   132, 262
pyloric stenosis   192–3
pyrexia, post-operative   260–3

raised intracranial pressure   46–7
Ranson criteria   103
red eye   176–8
renal colic see ureteric colic
renal failure, acute   59–61
renal stones   128–9
reperfusion therapies   15
replacement fluid regimes   156–7
    burn injuries   166–8
    paediatrics   200
    pre-eclampsia   209
respiratory arrest
    paediatric   197–9
    see also cardiopulmonary
        resuscitation
respiratory problems   2, 31–42
    asthma   31–4
    COPD   35–8
    pneumothorax   39–41, 154–5
    management principles   154–5
respiratory stimulants   37
restraint and de-escalation
        techniques   225–7
retinal detachment   180
retinopathy, hypertensive   27–8
retrobulbar haemorrhage   177
reversible ischaemic neurological
        deficit (RIND)   51
Reye's syndrome   243
rhabdomyolysis   64–5
RIND (reversible ischaemic
        neurological deficit)   51
Rovsing's sign   100
ruptured abdominal aortic
        aneurysms   134–5

SAFE approach   1
salicylate poisoning   241–3

sedation, and psychosis   226
seizures   56–8
    and eclampsia   210
self harm and suicide   228–30
sepsis   253–7
    multi-organ failure/dysfunction
        (MOF/DS)   106, 255–7
septic shock   253
septicaemia   253
sequestration crisis   92
shock   250–2
shoulder dystocia   213–14
sickle-cell crisis   91–3
sinus bradycardia   22–4
SIRS (systemic inflammatory response
        syndrome)   253–5
small bowel obstruction   117
spinal injuries   143–4
Staphylococcus aureus
    infections   218–19
    MRSA   253
status epilepticus   56–8
Stevens Johnson's syndrome   173–5
strangulated hernia   117, 119–20
streptococcal infections   220
stridor   187–9
stroke   51–3
subarachnoid haemorrhage   54–5
subdural haemorrhage   54–5
suicide and self-harm   228–30
superior vena caval (SVC)
        obstruction   97–8
supraventricular tachycardia
        (SVT)   17–18, 20
SVC (superior vena caval)
        obstruction   97–8
SVT (supraventricular
        tachycardia)   17–18, 20
Synacthen test   79
systemic inflammatory response
        syndrome (SIRS)   253–5

tachycardia
    broad complex   20–1
    narrow complex   17–19
    and shock   251
tamponade, cardiac   9, 29–30

TB meningitis   48–50
tension pneumothorax   9, 39–40,
      154
testicular torsion   126–7
tetanus risk   170
thoracic injuries   154–5
thrombolysis   15, 85, 139
thrombosis
      acute limb ischaemia   139–40
      deep vein   81–2
tonic–clonic seizures   56–8
toxic epidermal necrolysis
      (TENS)   173
toxic megacolon   115
toxic shock syndrome (TSS)   218–20
      staphylococcal infections
            218–19
      streptococcal infections   220
TRALI (transfusion-associated lung
      injury)   96
tranquillisation   226
transfusion reactions   94–6
transient ischaemic attacks
      (TIAs)   51
trauma
      airways   152–3
      breathing   154–5
      circulation   156–7
      general principles   149
      paediatrics   199–200
      primary survey   149–50
      secondary survey   150
tricyclic antidepressant
      overdose   246–9

ulcerative keratitis   177
umbilical cord prolapse   211–12
unstable angina   13–14
upper gastrointestinal
      bleeding   121–3
ureteric colic   128–9
urinary alkalinisation   242–3
urinary tract infection (UTI)   262
urine retention   130–1

Valsalva manoeuvre   17
vaso-occlusive crisis   91
ventricular fibrillation (VF)   5–7
      paediatrics   199
ventricular tachycardia (VT)   5,
      20–1
violent patients, and psychosis
      225–7
vision loss   179–81
      age-related macular
            degeneration   181
      central retinal artery
            occlusion   179
      central retinal vein
            occlusion   179–80
      ischaemic optic neuropathy
            180
      retinal detachment   180
      vitreous haemorrhage   180
vitreous haemorrhage   180

Wood's screw manoeuvre   214
wounds   169–70
      infections   260–1